A Concise Handbook
of Community Psychiatry
and Community Mental Health

Edited by
Leopold Bellak, M.D.

Visiting Professor of Psychiatry,
Albert Einstein College of Medicine;
Research Professor of Psychology,
Postdoctoral Program in Psychotherapy,
New York University, New York, N.Y.;
Clinical Professor of Psychiatry and Behavioral Sciences,
George Washington School of Medicine,
Washington, D.C.

Grune & Stratton
A Subsidiary of Harcourt Brace Jovanovich, Publishers
New York and London

Library of Congress Cataloging in Publication Data

Bellak, Leopold, 1916-

A concise handbook of community psychiatry and
community mental health.

Includes bibliographical references.
1. Community mental health services—United States.
2. Social psychiatry—United States. I. Title.
[DNLM: 1. Psychiatry, Community. WM30 B435c 1974]
RA790.6.B46   362.2'2'0973   74-6249
ISBN 0-8089-0833-2

Grune & Stratton, Inc.
111 Fifth Avenue
New York, New York 10003

Library of Congress Catalog Card Number 74-6249
International Standard Book Number 0-8089-0833-2
Printed in the United States of America

To the spirit of John F. Kennedy
and to
The National Institute of Mental Health,
which has contributed so much to my own work and to
research, training, and service in the mental health field.
With loyalty and appreciation
in these years of darkness and with the hope
that before too long a return of Enlightenment
will again permit me to quarrel with personalities
and policies at NIMH for constructive ends

Contents

Foreword   *Erich Lindemann, M.D., Ph.D.*   ix

Acknowledgments   xi

Contributors   xiii

Overview and Introduction:
Community Mental Health—10 Years Later   *Leopold Bellak*   1

PART I   Meeting Community Mental Health Center Problems

1   A Multimodality Continuous Care Program
in the Bronx   *Israel Zwerling*   15

2   Two Models for Organizing Mental Health Care
Delivery   *William Goldman*   31

3   A Suburban Clinic in Transition   *Harvey H. Barten*   43

4   An Experiment in District Psychiatry in Paris:
Psychiatry for the Community and in the Community
Serge Lebovici and Philippe Paumelle   69

**PART II   Current Special Problems and Special Services
in Community Mental Health**

5   Old Age   *Nathan Sloate*   91

6   Childhood   *Irving N. Berlin*   105

7   Drug Abuse   *Herbert D. Kleber*   129

8   Alcoholism   *Morris E. Chafetz*   163

PART III   Beyond the Community Mental Health Center

9   Toward Health Maintenance Organization
     Robert L. Leopold   183

10   A Nonmedical Model for Community Mental Health
     John C. Glidewell   205

11   Policy Aspects of Citizen Participation
     William M. Bolman   219

     Index   243

Foreword

This Handbook is composed of a number of stimulating contributions which show the far-flung parameters of the field in which mental health issues occur. The goals are no longer limited to health and disease, but include guiding each person to the most acceptable and achievable life-style of which he might be capable. Instead of dealing mainly with patients, or potential patients, the most significant interaction takes place with persons in the community who make decisions about mental health arrangements, and carry out the numerous new roles which seem to be required by preventive programs.

Events are moving quickly in this field, and at this point in history it begins to be possible to make some inferences from recent experience: from some successes and from many failures. The community mental health centers are the expression of a powerful ideological thrust which had its origins in psychiatry and public health and which was fostered by the intellectual climate of the Kennedy period. Overextension of goals, improvised planning, collision with existing power structures, and inevitable retrenchment on many fronts are recurrent themes which arise in the editor's introductory statement, and are encountered again and again in the more specific contributions of well-chosen experts. It was wise and courageous to take stock in this form of the almost chaotic features of the developing community mental health program, while making abundantly clear the encouraging discoveries and methodological advances which have emerged and are continuing to appear. The book will be helpful reading for a wide range of professionals, scholars, and citizens.

Erich Lindemann, M.D., Ph.D.
Clinical Professor of Psychiatry,
Stanford University School of Medicine, Stanford, California;
Professor of Psychiatry Emeritus, Harvard University, Cambridge, Massachusetts

Acknowledgments

I am very grateful to Ann Noll for editorial help, especially with the beginnings of the book and most specifically for bringing her expertise to bear in the chapter on alcoholism; to Rhoda Katzenstein for work on various chapters and especially on the editing of Chapter 4; and to Caroline Birenbaum for overseeing editorial problems of the final phase of the volume. Caryl Snapperman as editor at Grune & Stratton was a pleasure to cooperate with.

L. B.

Contributors

Harvey H. Barten, M.D., Clinical Associate Professor, Cornell Medical College, New York, New York; Medical Director, The Guidance Center of New Rochelle, New Rochelle, New York

Irving N. Berlin, M.D., Professor of Psychiatry and Pediatrics; Head, Division of Child Psychiatry, University of Washington, Seattle, Washington

William M. Bolman, M.D., Professor of Psychiatry, University of Hawaii School of Medicine, Honolulu, Hawaii

Morris E. Chafetz, M.D., Director, National Institute of Alcohol Abuse and Alcoholism, Rockville, Maryland

John C. Glidewell, Ph.D., Professor of Education, Department of Education, University of Chicago, Chicago, Illinois

William Goldman, M.D., Commissioner, Department of Mental Health, Commonwealth of Massachusetts; formerly Executive Director, Westside Community Mental Health Center, Inc., San Francisco, California

Herbert D. Kleber, M.D., Associate Professor of Clinical Psychiatry, Yale University School of Medicine; Director, Drug Dependence Unit, Connecticut Mental Health Center, New Haven, Connecticut

Serge Lebovici, M.D., Professor of Child Psychiatry, University of Paris VI; Director, Child Mental Health Center, 13th arrondissement, Paris, France

Robert L. Leopold, M.D., Professor and Chairman, Department of Community Medicine, University of Pennsylvania, Philadelphia, Pennsylvania

Philippe Paumelle, M.D., Director, Adult Mental Health Center, 13th arrondissement, Paris, France

Nathan Sloate, Special Assistant to the Director, National Institute of Mental
Health, Rockville, Maryland

Israel Zwerling, M.D., Ph.D., Chairman, Department of Mental Health
Sciences, Hahnemann Medical College, Philadelphia, Pennsylvania; formerly
Director, Bronx State Hospital, Bronx, New York

Leopold Bellak, M.D.

Overview and Introduction: Community Mental Health— 10 Years Later

The publishers asked me to revise the *Handbook of Community Psychiatry* which appeared in 1964.[1] I soon found that in the roughly 10 years since its inception the field of community psychiatry and community mental health had changed so drastically that there was no point in revising in the sense of updating the material in the previous volume. A totally new book was necessary.

10 YEARS OF EVOLUTION

Some of the issues which were urgent in the early 1960s have been resolved to a satisfactory extent. For instance, training in community psychiatry is a well-established discipline taught in many centers. Also, mental health consultation and the use of general hospitals for psychiatric patients are now matters of course. If any state hospitals have not been reorganized along more enlightened lines, it is not for lack of know-how.

On the other hand, areas and issues in community mental health about which we then knew little have clearly emerged as the most urgent problems today. Among these are some to which whole chapters are devoted in this volume: the three As—addiction, alcoholism, aging—and the still insufficiently appreciated problem of community mental health services for children. Existing services need to be rendered in more sophisticated ways, as continuous care but of widely differing nature, as the first four chapters of the present volume discuss. Finally, there is the question whether community psychiatry and community mental health go far enough or whether integration into even more comprehensive social planning isn't essential for headway in the mental health field. The health mobilization organization (HMO) and even broader schemes are attempts in that direction and are discussed later.

1

In the 1964 *Handbook* I suggested that community psychiatry might be seen as the third revolution, the age of enlightenment being the first and the advent of Freud and psychoanalysis the second. While the term is widely used now, some including myself have suggested that it would be better to speak of "evolution" rather than "revolution."

Conceptually I believe evolution is a better term, and I will address myself to it. But what I caught in speaking of the third revolution was that the concept of community mental health involved a certain revolutionary spirit and zest which today survives mainly in some of the neighborhood crisis-intervention centers in ghettos—and is at times, in fact, misplaced.

It was in February 1963 that President John F. Kennedy sent a message to Congress outlining the Community Mental Health Act. Congress adopted it in October 1963. It was part of Camelot.

Underlying the community mental health approach was an ideology which, because it was implicit and not conscious, was often all the more an important determinant and direct offspring of the spirit of enlightenment. To the extent that help was being offered to the disadvantaged of the community, a liberal ideology facilitated the desire to extend care for mental health to include help with problems of an economic, racial, and cultural nature. For this service, even with the best intentions, neither the mental health workers nor their center were equipped, nor were adequate funds available. At times, in fact, mental health centers and activities were embroiled in the political strife of a community—both the community and the mental health services suffering for it, but growing with it.

The same revolutionary zeal made community mental health often a movement rather than a discipline: To the extent that mental patients themselves had indeed been disenfranchised by commitment procedures and poor care in custodial institutions, their cause became another anti-Establishment cause with often far-reaching and overreaching consequences. The very concept of psychoses was changed by the community mental health concept, both for better and for worse.

The fact is that community mental health, like most if not all sciences, but certainly like all treatment modalities, went through certain phases, the first of which I have elsewhere called the *heroic phase*. An individual drug or a particular therapeutic modality in its initial phase seems to be an answer to virtually all problems, and previous modalities seem outmoded, devalued, and to be discarded. After this initial enthusiastic thesis, some flaws are found, the limitations become obvious, and some people begin as an antithesis to discredit that entire therapeutic modality. If all goes well, and if there was any substance at all to the discovery, this phase of relative disenchantment is followed by a third phase, that of synthesis, wherein the useful aspects become so integrated with the rest of the field of knowledge that they are soon taken for granted and barely noticed, while some other new magic discovery enjoys the limelight. These Hegelian phases can easily be identified in the development of psychoanalysis as well as in the history of psychotropic drugs.

In the heroic phase of community mental health of these past 10 years, hundreds of mental health centers have been established across these United States, accompanied by such satellites as neighborhood intervention centers, affiliated agencies, consultation services, and other programs.

State hospitals have changed from authoritarian institutions of horror to usually enlightened facilities with trained personnel and relatively few residual long-term patients, and with a variety of treatment modalities. The private sector of the economy has participated via some often quite liberal insurance coverages and the comprehensive medical care policies of larger corporations.

In the heroic phase (when community psychiatry was considered an answer to virtually all problems in the field) some attitudes were as reasonable as if somebody had discovered the field of public health and thereupon decided that the study of anatomy, physiology, and pharmacology were no longer necessary, and that widespread use of epidemiological principles of water supply and sewage disposal made specialties such as cardiology and surgery unnecessary. In the heroic phase of community mental health, the need for clinical training in any of the individual disciplines—social work, psychology, psychiatry—seemed not too relevant. So great was the interest in the quantity of care to be made available that concern with the quality of care suffered somewhat.

The fact that community mental health was defined as a method of care delivery was at the heart of the problem. In the earlier *Handbook* I suggested that community mental health could be defined as "the resolve to view the individual's problems of mental health within the frame of reference of the community" and vice versa. I regret that this suggestion never became popular. Instead, community mental health was described as "a system of mental health services delivered to the community." This concept, I believe, may have facilitated overemphasizing delivery and sometimes underemphasizing the product to be delivered. To a certain extent, what I once nastily wrote in response to an overenthusiastic (to my mind) report on Soviet psychiatry also holds true for some American community psychiatry. I suggested that Soviet community psychiatric services could be compared to an excellent postal system with nothing to deliver.[2]

Despite all the critical comments one can make about the development of community mental health, the field has made tremendous strides, and some early errors have been corrected.

Some slight statistical evidence for the trend toward emphasis on quantity over quality came from the decline of candidates for psychoanalytic training. This process has now clearly reversed itself. From first-hand experience, I know this does not mean that most of these young psychiatrists do not plan to work in community mental health. As far as I can see, most of them merely wish to acquire psychoanalytic skills, partly in order to have a better understanding of community psychiatric problems. This is one area where some synthesis in the field has been achieved.

In the heroic phase an attempt was made to abolish hospitalization altogether. It becomes clearer almost daily that this trend is being reversed toward a more reasonable synthesis of old and new ideas. For instance, the study of treatment of

psychotics in the home by Pasamanick and his associates[3] was awarded the Hof-
heimer Research Prize in 1961 by the American Psychiatric Association. However, the early enthusiasm of this study has now been decreased by a follow-up
study of Pasamanick's own, in which it appears that in the long run ''there were
no statistical, significant differences, among the groups on the extent of clinical
care received during the follow-ups. . . . Patients in all groups deteriorated on task
performance over time'' (p. 15).[4] That is, the ones treated in the hospital and
the ones treated in their own homes did equally well or equally poorly.

Part of this disappointment seems due to the heroic concept of community
mental health, which suggested that all severely ill psychotics could be treated
without hospitalization, that psychiatric patients could be depended upon to control
their own care and would continue to take prescribed medication and attend clinics,
or that their families would take the necessary responsibility. The last was an even
greater illusion than the others.

This concept—this misconception—of the nature of psychosis in the early
phase of community psychiatry ran its extreme course in the antipsychiatry movement which found adherents in Europe as well as in the United States. The main
exponents of this view held (1) that psychosis was a perfectly normal way of ad-
justing to our society and psychotics should be left alone to work out their own
problems, (2) that in fact psychotics were healthy and our society as a whole ill—a
painful view one can still sometimes feel sympathetic to, or (3) that psychiatry as
part of the Establishment was robbing the patient of his civil rights simply because
he didn't conform and that society insisted upon judging undesirable behavior as
pathological behavior. Conceptual confusion of goodwill with facts led such an
otherwise sound and responsible group as the New York Civil Liberties Union to
support attempts to abolish all commitment procedures as deprivation of civil
rights.

Even the best intentions can lead to evil results. New York's recent revision
of laws governing the care of the mentally ill were meant to strengthen the policy
of voluntary admission and easy discharge of patients. The *New York Times* properly questioned whether this move was toward freedom or hypocrisy:

> Compulsory custody is now limited to 15 days, and thousands will be turned loose to the
> hazards of a community which they cannot deal with and which does not provide halfway
> houses or other modalities which they could use. A mixture of good intentions and exces-
> sive zeal and a misconception of the nature of psychoses outrunning society's willingness
> to provide proper care is likely to lead to a worsening of the fate of psychotics.[5]

Despite some errors, we are on the way to synthesis between Establishment
control and antipsychiatry, so that some previously mistreated and terribly neglected psychiatric patients, who had indeed often been cruelly deprived of their
rights, now have better protection and are legally entitled to proper care instead
of being shut away as skeletons in closets—which huge state hospitals far away
from the community used to represent.

COMMUNITY PSYCHIATRY AND THE CONCEPT OF PSYCHOSIS

Having traced the evolution of the field and the concept of community psychiatry, let me turn to a few specific examples of the ways in which community psychiatry affected the concept of the psychoses.

Before a patient went to a state hospital 10 or 15 years ago, he was usually first placed in a receiving hospital, where in the absence of psychotropic drugs and facilities, he was frequently kept in wet packs, restraints, strong rooms. He was then shipped off, dehydrated and panic-stricken, after approximately 10 days, to a state hospital 20–50 miles away from where he lived, accessible only with great difficulty and infrequently by a few relatives who cared enough to make the effort. These state hospitals usually housed from 2000 to 10,000 patients, with often a ratio of 500 patients to 1 doctor. In essence, the patients were forced into a situation resembling experimental conditions of *perceptual isolation*. They sat shabby-clothed day in and day out in long corridors.

One must consider the possibility that the typical chronic or extreme features of the schizophrenic syndrome were *iatrogenic:* if not physician-induced directly, then certainly induced by the so-called medical management of the patients. Under the impact of forced isolation, lack of motivation, and lack of any social functioning, many of the patients' ego functions regressed. This accounted not only for complete apathy, but also for deterioration of at least some of the ego functions, thus facilitating bizarre delusions and hallucinations. I want to emphasize that the whole concept of deterioration in schizophrenia has to be newly examined in the light of changes wrought by community mental health, beyond the original dialogue between the Kraepelinian and the Bleulerian viewpoints. Deterioration in schizophrenia may have little to do with the disorder or syndrome per se, but may rather be a form of *disuse atrophy of ego functions*, produced by the enforced schizophrenic way of life in custodial institutions. Features considered typical of chronic schizophrenia, such as trichotillomania (the tendency to pull out, and often eat, one's own hair) may reflect, aside from regression, a stimulus hunger desperate to the point of inducing pain to provide stimulation, even by self-mutilation. The once widely practiced wrist slashing by breaking a pane of glass with the bare hand was an attempt to fight depersonalization, using acute pain as an organizing principle. Another phenomenon which was probably an artifact is Scheid's cyanotic syndrome, which often led to collapse and even death in acutely distrubed psychiatric patients, both manics and catatonics. It is extremely likely that this syndrome was the result not of any toxic condition as part of the psychotic process, but rather of exhaustion and excessive loss of electrolytes and fluids, which replacement can usually remedy.

Community psychiatry and drug therapy have changed the concept of psychosis with regard to these extreme and chronic manifestations. Today's psychiatric resident is no more likely to see catatonia with waxy flexibility than the medical resident is likely to see the four stages of pneumonia. Psychotropic drugs and antibiotics have altered the course long before the patient arrives at these stages.

A seemingly logical extension of the ability to change the nature of acute and chronic psychosis led to the notion that psychotics should be treated entirely like other people, and after cessation of the acute symptoms could simply be redischarged into the family and/or the community. The appropriate feeling that prior to community psychiatry the patient had been infantilized and forced to regress and the appropriate reversal of such policies were followed inappropriately by the concept that all patients could be easily reintegrated and that none needed long-term hospitalization. It was not understood that a vast percentage can at best tolerate only gradual transition into the community and need, at the very least, transitional modalities of living in the community-hotel wards, halfway houses, or other special communities. In the well-intentioned revolutionary zeal, it was easy to overlook some of these realities and to idealize the psychotic. One identified with the patient as underdog, and some came to think of the psychotic as "right" and the community as "wrong."

This thinking reminds me of some notions of Rousseau, whom I consider to be the father of the hippies and one of the first to be impressed with some undesirable features of technological civilization. He was led to admire primitive man and created the concept of the noble savage. Like the hip philosophy, this was an attempt to deal with the increasingly complex and vicious problems of interaction in our society by creating a fiction and attempting to turn back the clock. Elsewhere I have described the Rousseau delusion of the noble savage.[6] One could speak of the "noble psychotic" as a romantic and unrealistic concept of psychosis as a part of the heroic phase of community mental health. Rousseau, of course, had perceived perfectly accurately some of the evils of civilization. The fact that his picture of the noble savage was distorted does not imply that he may not have glimpsed quite correctly that technologically more primitive people had an ethnic culture and dignity of their own not at all consistent with "savagery."

Similarly, we know, that there is a logic to psychosis, a real human struggle with existence and attempts at problem solving in psychotic phenomena which often merit more appreciation than the indiscriminate swamping of all psychic functions with drugs. At the same time they hardly merit a romantic notion of a way of living or of problem solving superior to what the rest of us do with, by and large, more intact ego functions—of reality testing, judgment, sense of self, impulse control, object relations.

Let me enlarge specifically on some of the ill effects of this mistaken concept of psychosis on community mental health itself and on the community.

One must wonder how many professionals, more or less briefly in contact with their schizophrenic patients, are aware of the burden such a patient constitutes for the family unit. If one is engaged in intensive care of psychotics, one sees vividly how such families suffer from days and nights of acute upset on the part of the patient. The patient may threaten violence or suicide, may be actively deluded or hallucinated, may be sleepless, demanding, oversensitive, and noncontributory to the ordinary running of the household. The relatives of such a patient can live only with their emotions—an echo awakened in them pulling and tugging on regulation and control of impulses, and this appeals to their own primary processes so that anxiety and anger are aroused.

Berman relates the situation described so well in Goffman's essay, "The Insanity of Place." The enlightened psychiatrist wants to keep the patient home, but home life is now transformed:

'Households can hardly be operated if the goodwill of the residents cannot be relied on.' If the family must now stand guard duty, its normal forms of activity and division of labor will be wrecked. Now, anytime [the patient] picks up a knife, answers the phone, disappears from view, 'the family will have to be ready to jump.' Any object in the house may at any moment become an instrument with which he may harm others or himself. This ominous possibility can 'unhinge the meaning of domestic acts' for the whole family.[7]

Anthony and his associates[8] report that acutely disturbed schizophrenic parents seem to have a more disorganizing effect on children than relatively chronic, quiet schizophrenics. Clinical observation makes me believe that the siblings of schizophrenics are frequently overconstricted people. As one of them said in response to projective techniques: "I don't want to say anything that sounds crazy." There is an excessive need for rigid defenses and regulation and control of drives, and a great deal of anxiety.

In a controlled study conducted by Landau et al.[9] many interesting conclusions were formulated about the personality development of children raised by one or more psychotic parents. After careful experimentation, using a research and a control group, the workers found a definite delay in speech (and later, thought) development, more apparent stress and neglect, and more aggression and difficulty in forming interpersonal relationships with peers among the research group. These are only a few of the numerous differences this study revealed.

Less clear, but needing careful investigation, is what effect, if any, the presence of more or less acutely disturbed schizophrenics have on the village, the town, and the city in which they live. It may well turn out that they have no significant effect or at least no deleterious effect on the community at large.

Keeping psychotics in their communities, within their families, may show up advantageously as dollars saved on hospital maintenance. It will not be easily apparent, however, just how much the health, working ability, and creativity of various family members is impaired by having psychotics living at home.* It is entirely possible that the increase of active psychotics in the family and the commun-

---

*A study performed in Manchester, England, by Dr. Julius Hoenig and Marion W. Hammerson attempted to assess the burden on the families of schizophrenics. With a total sample of 102 patients, these workers recorded the complete effects, such as loss of earnings, changes in the lives of the other members of the household because of the illness, separation from children, and the presence of certain disturbing elements, such as noisiness and wandering around at night. They called a total of 30 variables "the combined objective" burden on the family and concluded that it existed in 84 percent of their patients' cases; only 16 percent of the households did not seem affected in any of the 30 ways. The researchers seemed to note that patients who had been in a general hospital were less of a burden to the family than those who had been in a mental hospital. It is unclear from the report whether this might not be a result of lesser illness in those capable of being cared for in a general hospital.[10]

ity may lead to a *mental health pollution* much as technological progress increases ecological pollution.

SOME ARTIFACTS OF COMMUNITY PSYCHIATRY

Other problems related to community psychiatry are emerging. For example, "in Suffolk County on Long Island, where six large mental institutions exist, more than 5,000 of the 60,000 . . . on welfare are former patients of state mental institutions."[11] The problem is the same in other counties where large mental institutions are situated. As the treatment of mental patients is shifted from state hospitals to the community, patients are more or less dumped onto the community.

Many of the contemplated community mental health clinics have not been built or have not been staffed and are unable to care for the discharged patients. Most patients do not return voluntarily for aftercare. Some who have been on wards with a completely controlled life are turned loose into rooming houses. In one instance in the town of Bayshore on Long Island, 60 patients living in a crowded frame building were "frequently found wandering across neighbors' lawns in the middle of the night. Several appeared on the main thoroughfare [of the town] directing traffic." Others, one doctor was quoted in the *New York Times*, "are walking the streets of Manhattan: many of the derelicts and alcoholics in New York City who sleep in the doorways at night and panhandle in the daytime were formerly patients at Central Islip Hospital" (p. 59).[11]

Another problem is quite clearly that the communities have not been sufficiently prepared for accepting patients into their midst. Frequently communities protest against halfway houses and other community mental health facilities.

The fact is that specific techniques must be developed for estimating patients' potential for psychosocial adjustment. At present, according to the National Institute of Mental Health,[8] only 15–40 percent of schizophrenics living in the community achieve what might be termed an average level of adjustment, i.e., are self-supporting or successfully functioning as a housewife.

Some practices of community psychiatric treatment remind me of the farmer who tried to accustom his donkey to living without food: He gave it a little less to eat each day and just when he seemed to succeed, the donkey died. Some people in the field seem to think that schizophrenia will disappear if we ignore it, or at any rate, if we do as little as possible for the patients. Surely, excessive hospitalization and excessive seclusion are bad for the schizophrenic—and for other people as well. That does not mean that no or minimal hospitalization is good for all schizophrenics—even though it may be good for some schizophrenics under optimal community care.

We are all familiar with one undesirable result of current therapeutic practice, compounded in equal parts of drug treatment and community psychiatry. The revolving-door phenomenon is the name of the game, and the fact is that while in the last 15 years the number of patients in hospitals at a given time has dec-creased by 15 percent, in the same time, the readmission figures have risen tremen-ously. In the United States, the probability of readmission within 2 years is be-tween 40 and 60 percent; between 15 and 25 percent of patients are eventually readmitted for continued long-term care.

One effect of this revolving-door phenomenon is the repeated integration of the patient into the community. This repetition suggests a need for reconsideration of our patient care and reflects to a certain extent a failure of community psychiat-ric therapy and of drug therapy. In order to keep, as well as treat, the patients in the community, we have to develop specific programs for them. We cannot naively discharge them into the community and vaguely expect that "community mental health facilities" will see them through.

FUTURE DIRECTIONS

In conclusion, hoping that despite current government policy there will still be some community mental health centers left to improve, I can only point to the programs described later in this volume: the sectorization of the 13th arrondisse-ment in Paris; the multiphasic, multimodal, continuous care program at Bronx State Hospital; the mental health consortia in Detroit, Chicago, San Francisco, and Los Angeles; and the prospective trend toward health mobilization organizations and HEW satellites, if state funding ever allows development of programs.

A special interest of mine is to insist upon the need for more accurate assess-ment of the assets and liabilities of each individual, and the tailoring of treatment programs including eventual disposition with regard to the best modality of living. My own preference has been to examine carefully the status of 12 ego functions and to arrive at a profile (the result of 5 years of research) which I believe can be used as a relatively experimentally verifiable method, as well as a good prag-matic clinical guideline, as I have described in a number of publications and in a recently published book. [12-15]

Beyond the care concept of psychosis, the consideration of social, as well as medical and experiential psychodynamic, problems as HEW satellites might do, makes good sense. As long as poverty and overcrowding exist, I doubt that the best psychiatric approach will reverse, let alone prevent, serious psychiatric problems. A special socioeconomic phenomenon related to psychiatric problems is the higher percentage of precipitate births among the poor. With such births goes a much higher proportion of the minimal brain syndrome, which causes primary disorders such as dyslexia, neurological difficulties with self-image, and problems of perceptual rela-tion to the environment, as well as secondary emotional problems which relate to serious psychiatric illness, including schizophrenia.

To the extent that other medical conditions, such as early encephalitic episodes, may predispose to later psychiatric disorder, medical care must be a part of the planning for community mental health and vice versa. If heredity is indeed shown to be responsible for at least a certain percentage of psychoses, genetic counseling will have to play an increasing role.

THE CONTEMPORARY SCENE

It is not enough merely to hope for a rational model of psychosis or a working model of community mental health. Neither will be produced if we remain only community mental health workers, psychologists, social workers, psychiatrists. They will develop only if we are an integral part of the political action to implement these programs.

The policy of the current national administration poses special problems for all aspects of the nation's health, welfare, and education. The cuts in appropriation for most mental health programs will do some irreparable harm to the patients and the workers, at least for the foreseeable future. Aside from this hardship imposed by decreased funds for a large number of services, the field is specifically affected by decreased chances for research and training. The most disastrous effect of administration policy on mental health may well be caused by the closing out of career research and training fellowship programs in psychiatry. They seem to have been the most fruitful venture in the mental health field of the last decade. With the help of these programs, young psychiatrists had a chance to be exposed to sophisticated centers of research where they learned the methodology, concept formation, and statistical thinking which medical schools and psychiatric residencies could not provide. Because of this acquired understanding, these Fellows seemed to me a nucleus of advancing sophistication in the field. They provided a welding of clinical, experimental, and academic skills, of psychiatry and psychology and other sciences. I see no way of avoiding the catastrophic effects of the abolition of these programs.

The effects of this deprivation and lack of preventive services will be felt in coming years. However, the imposed austerity may just possibly have some constructive effects.

In my introduction to a volume on contemporary European psychiatry,[16] I compared cultural matrixes and achievements of American and European psychiatry. I suggested that European psychiatry had produced virtually all the major advances and ideas in the field, even excluding Freud and other pre-World War II contributions. Electric convulsive therapy, Metrazol, insulin, chlorpromazine, reserpine, and almost the whole field of psychotropic drugs (lately including lithium from Australia) came primarily from Europe. Use of lysergic acid diethylamide for the study of model psychoses came from Europe; so did community mental health—largely from Britain and Holland.

I suggested a possible connection between the economic condition of European psychiatry and its creativity, and the American economy and its lack of creativity (without denigrating the great methodological and organizational implementation in the United States). Two factors may have played a role in European creativity. First, the need to work out problems with string and paste and individual work rather than oversophisticated instruments may have the same effect on research creativity as painstaking tilling of a small piece of land has on agricultural productivity compared with mass-production processes. Second, the much smaller opportunity for advancement and mobility from one situation to another may have provided a better milieu for creativity. In the American setting, a successful bright young psychiatrist who has made any kind of contribution promptly moves on to another institution, a higher salary, and often a higher position. His work is interrupted and his eye is on the next chance for betterment. Soon he is an important administrator without creative research activity. One need only peruse journals to find that a piece was written at one institution, the work done at a previous institution, and the author at present affiliated with yet another center!

I do not wish to preach the virtues of poverty or to imply that budgetary cuts are likely to have anything but primarily destructive effects on service, training, and research. However, while we are in this period of budgetary disaster, we may possibly profit from it by adaptation to this crisis, as to any other crisis. Instead of being absorbed in acquiring more buildings and having more staff and money for large collaborative teams, we can try to make existing services qualitatively better and more effective. We can spend more time thinking creatively. Staff and chairmen of departments might spend more time at their own desks or laboratories than as guests at some distant institution. This might limit cross-fertilization, but increase fertility at home.

One must hope that political enlightenment and economic balance will soon permit again the spirit of American enlightenment which found its expression in the Community Mental Health Act and other progressive social legislation. Let us work toward this goal. But meanwhile, let us make productive use of the limited advantages of adversity.

REFERENCES

1. Bellak L: Handbook of Community Psychiatry. New York, Grune & Stratton, 1964
2. Bellak L: The role of psychoanalysis in contemporary psychiatry. Am J Psychother 24:470–476, 1970
3. Pasamanick B, Scarpatti F, Dinitz S: Schizophrenics in the Community: An Experimental Study in the Prevention of Hospitalization. New York, Appleton, 1967
4. Grant HM: Long term progress seen as bleak for schizophrenics. Psychiatric News, Dec 6, 1972, p 15
5. Freedom or hypocrisy. New York Times, Feb 7, 1973, p 38
6. Bellak L: The Porcupine Dilemma. New York, Citadel Press, 1970
7. Berman M: Relations in public. New York Times Book Review, Feb 27, 1973, p 16
8. National Institute of Mental Health, Center for Studies in Schizophrenia: Special Report: Schizophrenia. Publication No (HSM) 72-9007. Rockville, Md, U.S. Department of Health, Education and Welfare, 1971
9. Landau R, Harth P, Othnay N, Scharfhertz C: The influence of psychotic parents on their children's development. Am J Psychiatry 129:1, 1972
10. Reaction of family studied in schizophrenics' home care. Psychiatric News, Aug 15, 1973, p 22
11. Andelman DA: Discharged mental patients create problems in state. New York Times, Feb 13, 1972, pp 1 and 59
12. Bellak L, Hurvich M: Ego function patterns in schizophrenics. Psychol Rep 22:229–308, 1968
13. Bellak L, Hurvich M: A systematic study of ego functions. Ment Dis 148:569–585, 1969
14. Bellak L, Hurvich M, Gediman H, Craw-

ford PJ: A study of ego functions in the
schizophrenic syndrome. Arch Gen Psychiatry 23:326–336, 1970

15.   Bellak L, Hurvich M, Gediman H: Ego
Functions in Schizophrenics, Neurotics,
and Normals, New York, John Wiley and
Sons, 1973

16.   Bellak L (ed): Contemporary European
Psychiatry. New York, Grove Press, 1961

PART I

Meeting Community Mental Health Center Problems

Israel Zwerling, M.D., Ph.D.

1

A Multimodality Continuous Care Program in the Bronx

In the presidential address to the American Psychiatric Association in 1958, Harry C. Solomon stated:

> The large mental hospital is antiquated, outmoded, and rapidly becoming obsolete. We can still build them but we cannot staff them; and therefore we cannot make true hospitals of them. After 114 years of effort, in this year 1958, rarely has a state hospital an adequate staff as measured against the minimum standards set by our Association . . . and these standards represent a compromise between what was thought to be adequate and what it was thought had some possibility of being realized. . . . I do not see how any reasonably objective view of our mental hospitals today can fail to conclude that they are bankrupt beyond remedy. I believe therefore that our large mental hospitals should be liquidated as rapidly as can be done in an orderly and progressive fashion.[1]

The processes which, starting in the latter half of the 19th century, had rendered the large mental hospitals into underfinanced, understaffed, geographically isolated custodial warehouses have been described,[2] and their explication lies outside the central concern of this report. What is of present relevance is that a reaction to the shame of these hospitals was without question a significant component in the confluence of forces which led to the explosive development of community psychiatry programs in the late 1950s. An explicitly stated goal of such programs was, precisely, the liquidation of mental hospitals.

The development of community-based inpatient and outpatient alternatives to the state mental hospitals has indeed brought about dramatic changes in the care and treatment of psychotic patients. The principal locus of treatment has increasingly been the community facility rather than the mental hospital; in New York State, for example, the average daily census in state hospitals has fallen from 92,165 in 1955 to 38,515 in October, 1973. The career of a model patient has been altered, from long-term or even lifetime institutionalization punctuated by

15

brief stays in the community, to long-term community residence punctuated by brief periods of hospitalization. Although many intertwined factors, perhaps most notably the antipsychotic drugs, have concurrently been operative, it is ultimately the availability of community resources as alternatives to hospitalization which has made this transition possible. At the same time, it is becoming increasingly evident that there are risks inherent in the mushrooming of community programs which may threaten the goals of shifting treatment from the hospital to the community for some patients, particularly the chronically psychotic, alcoholic, addicted, and elderly patients.

It has been noted[3] that community mental health centers have tended to focus attention, in the main, on patients with acute psychoses, neuroses, and personality disorders, and on those problems of coping with the stresses of daily living which are related more to improving the quality of life than to remedying chronic mental disability. The referral flow of patients for treatment options between the mental hospital and the community mental health center tends to be unidirectional, from the center to the hospital, with only referrals for aftercare of discharged patients flowing from the hospital to the community facility, and then only when the latter elects or is mandated to provide aftercare. In what frequently emerges as a competition between hospitals and community facilities for patients most likely to respond to currently available treatment regimens, the mental health centers enjoy many advantages. University and teaching hospital departments of psychiatry are increasingly utilizing community mental health centers in their teaching and training programs; unless they happen to be located in the vicinity of a mental hospital, the trainee and teaching staffs of these departments are unlikely to follow patients into the public mental hospital. The community mental health centers then, given first contact with patients, with substantial teaching obligations, and generally with better financial support than mental hospitals, tend to treat selectively the "good teaching cases"—precisely the patients we already are best able to treat. The state hospital, ringed by mental health centers, can then expect only those patients who are least likely to respond to current treatment approaches. Hospital staff members interested in active treatment may tend, as a consequence, to be attracted to the mental health centers, and this process, once begun, can develop its own momentum so that a rapid sorting out of professional staff may be expected. It is thus likely in some instances that community mental health centers, designed in large part to reverse the tendency of large mental hospitals to promote chronicity in mentally ill patients, will themselves become significant forces for promoting chronicity.

This pattern of patient flow is not entirely without significant advantages. The flexibility in selectively addressing community needs which the newly created centers require is maximized by having the mental hospitals as a captive backstop. The hospitals at the same time serve as reservoirs of professional manpower for the centers. Geographical distances between centers and hospitals are no deterrent to this pattern; indeed, the extrusion of undesired patients from community mental health centers is promoted by greater distances between the centers and the state hospitals. However, the promotion of chronicity and the building in of discontinuity between community and hospital phases of treatment seem much too steep a price to pay for these advantages.

An alternative model is one in which the mental hospital serves as the regional hub of a network of community-based mental health centers, with each geographical unit of the hospital fully integrated into the network of services designed for a defined catchment area or serving itself as the principal locus of a community mental health center. The essence of this model is a regionalization of mental health services around the unitized mental hospital, in close parallel to the catchment area subregions served by community mental health centers. Liaison patterns are then developed which involve the flow of patients between a hospital and a center, rather than exclusively between a center and the agencies and institutions in the community served by the center. It is the purpose of this report to describe such a program.

A prefatory caveat must be entered concerning the difficulty of evaluating this, or any, program concerned with the treatment of chronically psychotic patients. First, the criteria which immediately present themselves—readmission rates, duration of hospitalization during exacerbations of illness—are highly sensitive to a host of factors unrelated to the condition of the patient. For example, if few beds are available, and if outpatient alternatives do not exist or are inaccessible, readmission frequently serves as a solution to a crisis in community-based treatment. A large-scale natural experiment in the United States over the past quarter of a century illustrates this point sharply. The two largest states, California and New York, have approximately equal populations (19.9 million persons in the former, 18.2 million in the latter, in 1970). There are currently about 11,000 mental patients in hospitals in California, and about 50,000 in New York. This extraordinary discrepancy hardly reflects the advantages of the California climate. In the period immediately after World War II, both states invested substantially in expanding their mental health services. California developed an extensive network of outpatient clinics and filled all available places. New York built a network of large hospitals and filled all the beds. In some instances, inpatient services urge patients being discharged to return to the hospital on the occasion of the first faint evidences of difficulty, on the theory that it is more economical to have a larger number of brief admissions than a smaller number of extended admissions. The rate of rehospitalization, for these and other reasons, is an extremely unreliable index of the effectiveness of community treatment programs, and yet is probably the single most widely used criterion.

Second, it is evident that criteria based exclusively on the behavior and the fate of the identified patient do not take into account the burden placed on the family and community in extramural care of the patient. A family willing to replicate a hospital ward to retain one of its members at home can obviously keep a much sicker patient out of the hospital than can a family unwilling or incapable of tolerating any deviance in the behavior of the identified sick member. The more one studies families with a psychotic member, the clearer it becomes that at some juncture in family life the family—and not the admitting psychiatrist—makes the decision that the patient is to be returned to the mental hospital.

And finally, if a program is judged, by whatever criteria, to be successful in maintaining equilibrium in psychotic patients living in the community, the elements of the program responsible for its success cannot readily be sorted out because of the many variables at work. By the same token, no matter how carefully a successful program is described, it is virtually impossible to replicate it with precision in a new setting.

For all these reasons, the model of a regional hospital as the hub of a network of community-based long-term treatment facilities can be recommended only with caution, and conclusions drawn from the results observed must be held as tentative.

GENERAL DESCRIPTION

The programs described in this chapter are addressed—in by far the largest part—to an urban ghetto population which shares with the residents of Manhattan's Harlem and Brooklyn's Bedford-Stuyvesant sections leadership in every index of social pathology, including fiercely high rates of mental hospitalization. They are elements of a network of services in the Bronx—a county (or borough) of New York City, with approximately 1.5 million residents. The major facilities include the 1000-bed Bronx State Hospital; a children's psychiatric hospital currently staffed, because of budgetary restrictions, for 36 inpatients, but physically designed for 200; two community mental health centers, one with a 50-bed inpatient unit; two departments of psychiatry in municipal general hospitals, one with a 50-bed inpatient unit and the other with 12 beds; and three departments of psychiatry in voluntary general hospitals, one with 25 beds used principally for private patients, one with 14 beds used largely for indigent patients, and the third with only outpatient services. The Bronx State Hospital serves as the hub of the regional program for the care of chronically ill psychotic patients. It is "unitized," i.e., clusters of wards are organized as semiautonomous services or units, each devoted to a specific geographical area of the Bronx. Quite diverse liaison programs between the hospital services and community-based facilities exist, varying with the amount and quality of care and treatment provided by the latter facilities.

All the major psychiatric services in the Bronx are affiliated with the Albert Einstein College of Medicine. This is critical to an appreciation of the programs to be described. Much as is the case in the United Kingdom and in France, the administrative structure of public mental health services in New York State has built in a separation of the mental hospitals from the local community-based services at the very top, with a deputy commissioner responsible for each, and with functionally separate budgets supporting the hospitals on the one hand and the community-based services on the other. The result is an entirely predictable struggle between local and state-supported facilities about who is responsible for which patient. The principal factor which has made possible any success we may have enjoyed in developing liaison models has been the ultimate control of the executive committee and the chairman of the department of psychiatry of the medical school over the directors of each of the affiliated facilities. This is not an incidental point. If clusters of specialized facilities are administratively sequestered without responsibility to one overall regional authority, the possibility is that competitive, overlapping, and fragmented services rather than comprehensive and coordinated services will be available.

TREATMENT PROGRAMS AT BRONX STATE HOSPITAL

Confronted with psychotic behavior, one can answer the question, What's gone wrong? in one, two, or all of three general ways:

1. A neurobiological or neurochemical defect, inherited or acquired, has impaired basic mental processes—perception, memory, cognition, judgment—and has led to the psychotic behavior.
2. Psychological defects, conscious or unconscious, acquired early or late, and the consequence of real or fantasied traumas, are responsible for the production of abnormal dynamic sequences in adaptations to stress, conflict, frustration, or deprivation, including psychotic adaptations.
3. The psychosocial unit of which the psychotic person is a member—his family, community, or society—is governed by forces and counterforces so stressful and irrational that no suitable solution to basic problems, or no firm and secure membership in the unit, is possible for him, and the psychotic behavior is an understandable adaptation to the disturbed social matrix in which it is embedded.

It is not the intention here to suggest that one or another of these basic conceptual approaches to the cause of psychoses is to be preferred, or that they are indeed mutually exclusive. On the contrary, there is a growing consensus that all three explanatory hypotheses are relevant to any instance of psychotic behavior. Granted that one needs to be "wired"—anatomically or chemically—in such a manner as to be able to become psychotic, stress at the psychological or psychosocial level is required for the psychosis to become manifest. Conversely, no stress in itself can be demonstrated universally to result in psychosis. The approaches to treatment pursued by a hospital staff depend in part on the preferred explanation for psychotic behavior, and in part on available resources for intervention at the biological, psychological, or sociocultural levels of integration. At Bronx State Hospital, all three are represented.

Traditionally, the public mental hospital has been the arch-practitioner of organic therapies, and while insulin, lobotomy, carbon dioxide, and Metrazol have largely disappeared from the scene, electric convulsive therapy (ECT) and pharmacotherapy remain essential components of the treatment armamentarium of all but a small number of research hospitals. The impressive results in the treatment of psychotic depression with imipramine and amitriptyline have sharply reduced the use of ECT; Bronx State Hospital, for example, offers no ECT. The rather unusual patient with severe depression unresponsive to antidepressant medication for whom ECT is indicated is brought for treatment to the adjacent Bronx Municipal Hospital Center. Perhaps the most dramatic development in psychiatry in the past 15 years has been the elaboration of a spectrum of antipsychotic drugs, with variable but impressive effectiveness against psychotic excitement, paranoid ideation, and aggressive-assaultive behavior, with little impairment of cognitive functioning and with rather easily corrected side effects. Debates rage—and are likely to continue for some time—concerning the relative effectiveness of drugs versus psychotherapy versus sociotherapy, and concerning the relative effectiveness of drugs with or without other treatment. However, the effectiveness of drugs can hardly be challenged, and 90 percent of patients at Bronx State Hospital receive psychoactive drugs.

Psychotherapy may broadly be seen as either analytic-reconstructive, supportive, or reeducational in its goals and approach. The analytic-reconstructive model is based upon the premise that maladaptive behavior is the product of unconscious forces and counterforces within the mental apparatus of the individual patient. Intervention is then ideally intended, through clarification and the development of new insights into the thoughts, feelings, and actions of the patient, to bring these unconscious forces and counterforces into consciousness so that the full resources of the ego may be applied to the adaptational problems of everyday life. There is considerable doubt concerning the effectiveness of analytically oriented psychotherapy with psychotic patients. May[4] found psychotherapy the least effective and at the same time the most expensive form of treatment for hospitalized patients. Grinspoon et al.,[5] in a well-controlled double-blind study in which experienced therapists treated chronically schizophrenic patients, half of whom received placebos and half phenothiazines, found that after 2 years of intensive psychotherapy, there was no improvement in the placebo group whereas there was a significant reduction in psychotic symptomatology in the group receiving psychoactive drugs. Except for patients on the Tremont service of Bronx State Hospital, a unit operated by the psychiatric residents, virtually no patients are in intensive analytically oriented psychotherapy.

Supportive psychotherapy is a quite different kind of undertaking, sharing with analytically oriented psychotherapy only the property of attempting to effect behavioral change through psychological means. The disequilibrium between the conscious and unconscious forces and counterforces is approached here with the goal of strengthening conscious ego functions through a range of therapeutic strategies, including explanation, modeling, exhortation, approval, suggestion, and environmental change. The focus is on the here and now, rather than on the historical roots of present maladaptive behavior. The rationale is that a suitably buttressed ego structure can manage to effect viable compromises in all but a few extreme instances of intrapsychic or interpersonal conflicts. Virtually every patient at Bronx State Hospital is in a one-to-one therapeutic relationship with a supportive psychotherapist.

A special variant of supportive psychotherapy, based upon applications of conditioning theory and most widely referred to as "behavior modification," has recently been gaining increasing application, particularly but not exclusively from therapists trained in psychology. Rather than a general strengthening of ego functions, in the hope of providing adequate resources for managing previously disequilibrating conflicts, behavior modification is aimed in a highly specific way at the disabling symptoms of the patient. The rationale derives from the Skinnerian conditioning paradigm and the readily demonstrable effect of prompt rewards in increasing the frequency or intensity of desired behaviors. Through a combination of desensitization techniques, aimed at providing graduated exposure of the patient to unmanageable anxiety-provoking situations, and a system for rewarding adequate responses and punishing undesirable responses, the deviant behavior is gradually replaced by more adaptive behavior. Three wards at Bronx State Hospital operate token economy programs, in which patients' rewards (meals, cigarettes, home leaves) are contingent upon their receiving tokens in return for manifesting desired behaviors.

The organic and psychological therapies, despite their wide divergences in many fundamental respects, have in common the assumption that the state of mental illness is the product of a process taking place entirely within an individual. An alternative—not necessarily exclusive—assumption is that mental illness is a function of the processes of relatedness between and among human beings. The essential strategy in corrective intervention is then to provide paradigms for the critical social units—generally the family, but sometimes another or larger segment of the community—in which patients can be placed and opportunities for corrective experiences and for learning adaptational coping techniques can be provided. The general term for this treatment strategy, which attempts the creation of a therapeutic environment, is "milieu therapy," and perhaps the single most significant element in programs of milieu therapy is the "therapeutic community." The objective of such a unit, which consists of all participants—patients and staff alike—who live and/or work on a ward, is to establish a democratic community in which all members participate in decisions concerning life on the unit. Rather than the usual hierarchical ward structure in which patients are treated as though they lacked any capacity for making decisions for themselves, patients join with staff in regular meetings devoted to issues pertaining to the conduct of the business of the ward. On some wards, administrative policy dictates rather narrow limits to the range of the decision-making powers of the therapeutic community; in others, the widest latitude is given to the therapeutic community, including the decision to discharge patients. The theapeutic community approach is widely used at Bronx State Hospital. Our conviction is that if the range of issues confronted by a therapeutic community is sufficiently broad to ensure problems appropriate to all levels of competence among patients and staff members, in an unambiguous and honest community in which crises (or choices) are confronted and dealt with through open discussion and democratic process, ego growth cannot fail to occur.

A variety of sociotherapy which has recently stimulated considerable interest, and promises to open new directions for understanding mental illness, is "family therapy," i.e., psychotherapy in which the family as a unitary system is "the patient." The point is not merely to treat a patient in the presence of his family, although this may sometimes be of value in a program of individual psychotherapy, but to treat the family unit as the sick organism. The rationale for this approach is that the fundamental causative disequilibrium in mental illness is in the family system, and the identified patient is a manifestation of this disequilibrium, perhaps in the same way a swollen ankle may be a manifestation of cardiac or renal disease, or of hypoproteinemia, or of some other disturbance in the wider organismic system. The aim of the therapeutic intervention is to alter the system—its communications, its power relationships, its role distribution, its rules for relatedness among members, or whatever is perceived to be the crux of the disequilibrium. Bronx State Hospital has one of the largest training units in family therapy in the country. Recently this unit staffed a service assigned to a catchment area of 180,000 persons. The ward, day hospital, and outpatient clinic utilize all therapeutic modalities, but concentrate on family therapy as the principal treatment approach.

Activity group therapy, recreation therapy, and occupational therapy are sufficiently familiar modalities of sociotherapy to merit only passing mention. It is, however, worthy of note that to a significant degree the diversionary character of occupational therapy at Bronx State Hospital has given way to a work-for-pay program, a mode of industrial therapy which simulates as closely as possible reality work situations. The import of this trend derives from the broader shift toward shortening inpatient phases of treatment. The pressures of an inpatient service tend strongly to be centripetal, i.e., directed into the hospital. Even an outing of a group of patients and staff members of a hospital ward on a temporary visit to a museum or theater or bowling alley has the inescapable quality of a transient recreational venture out of and then back into the hospital. It has become apparent to us that a serious obstacle to the shortening of inpatient treatment programs is the attitude of hospital staff members that they must provide an asylum for "their" patients from the evil forces "out there" which made their charges ill, and that the hospital milieu must therefore be as different as possible from the "outside" world. The change in attitudes toward the recognition of the value to treatment of the greatest approximation of the hospital to the reality world of work and socialization has been slow in development. The growing number of centrifugal, community-directed sheltered workshop and industrial therapy programs, replacing the hospital-focused making of ashtrays and wicker baskets, is a healthy shift.

A final group of sociotherapies includes activities designed to stimulate intellectual and emotional growth. We have found art therapy, music therapy, and dance therapy useful adjuncts to treatment, in addition to serving as healthful elements of the hospital milieu. Dance therapy has made particularly impressive contributions, both through adding a rich store of nonverbal cues toward understanding the problems of patients and through imposing changes in motor patterns upon the behavioral profiles of tight, emotionally and physically rigid patients.

Bronx State Hospital thus offers a multimodality approach to treatment, including individual supportive psychotherapy, family and group therapy, drug therapy, milieu therapy, the creative arts therapies, and behavior modification therapy. It is, for the reasons proposed in the introductory section of this chapter, difficult to assess the relative effectiveness of the several approaches. It has been particularly striking to observe that, initially, each new effort (a token economy ward, a family studies ward, a group process ward) is an instant and dramatic success; the enthusiasm and morale of the staff translate into extraordinary efforts which, in turn, are reflected in the more rapid improvement of patients. An evaluation program is being developed which can take into account the many variables at work, and we hope to be able to contribute reliable data concerning the several treatment approaches being practiced.

A brief description of three special clinical programs will help round out a picture of the inpatient treatment services. First, since our patients inevitably include a number of women with preschool children, we have added training in mothering skills to the rehabilitation effort for these patients. Their children are admitted to a day nursery we operate, and the mothers spend part of their time taking turns with trained child-care workers in handling their children. In addition to our treatment and rehabilitation goals for the mothers, we see the children as a high-risk population for mental illness and hope to demonstrate a preventive effect of this effort.

Second, we accumulated a sizable population of mentally retarded adults who were transferred to Bronx State Hospital from state schools because of florid psychotic episodes the schools were not equipped to treat. We, in turn, had no program for this population of patients, once they were over the acute psychotic episode. No teachers with special education training are authorized to our hospital staff. Further, these patients were disruptive of ward treatment programs. They would, for instance, wander into and out of small group and therapeutic community meetings with no awareness of the ongoing activities. To deal with this especially difficult population, we organized a separate service, the cognitive development service, and designed specific programs (including a behavior modification program) for them. This unit has become one of the most exciting at our hospital. Within its first year of operation it had established a consultation center in a neighboring community which had no mental retardation services available.

Third, in an effort to correct too gross and empiric a use of psychoactive drugs, we established a psychopharmacology ward, designed to make precise observations of the behavioral effects of the neuroleptic agents in most common use. It has been heartening to see this unit begin to offer consultations to the other hospital services on medication problems and to conduct seminars on drug treatment.

RESIDENTIAL PROGRAMS

The gap between life as a patient on a hospital ward and life as a member of a fully independent household in a community is indeed great. The range of intermediary facilities which we have developed is incomplete, but does include some components which merit description.

To begin with, the hospital itself does not represent a sharp and total extrusion from family and community. It is located in the community. The wards are open. Visiting in the hospital is allowed every day, and patients are encouraged to spend evenings and weekends at home at the earliest feasible time. Deliberate efforts have been and are being made to encourage community use of the hospital grounds and facilities. Football and baseball fields have been provided without charge to a number of community organizations. The goal is that hospitalization should represent a hopefully brief move from one locus to another in the community.

As was noted above, therapeutic community programs within the hospital and the earliest use of day hospitalization are encouraged, in part to maximize the retention of responsibility for self and to minimize dependency and the loss of social skills. A particularly valuable predischarge residential component within the hospital which we have used extensively is the hotel ward, a ward operated with no, or token, staff, and where patients have full responsibility for taking medication, for organizing and implementing activity programs, and for leaving and returning to the hospital.

They see their therapist on schedule, much as though they were outpatients. If they voice physical complaints to referring ward staff members—an almost universal occurrence during the first day or two on an unsupervised ward—they are told they are free to call the medical clinic and make an appointment, much as they might call a neighborhood doctor when they are out of the hospital. In most such units, there are inadequate provisions for cooking for the entire hotel ward, so that patient groups take turns. Some cook, while others have regular hospital meals delivered to the ward.

Perhaps the most useful application of the hotel ward has been the opportunity provided to the staff to form small patient groups for discharge as units to our apartment program. Chronically ill patients notoriously are abandoned by their families. The problem of establishing a residence in the community for these patients is quite difficult; it is complicated by the shortage of low-cost apartments, by the reluctance of landlords to rent to tenants discharged from mental hospitals, and by the fear patients have of purchasing furniture and undertaking a long-term lease in the face of their experience of recurrent rehospitalizations. In order to deal with these problems we have utilized a nonprofit corporation which rents and furnishes apartments and leases them to discharged patients. They, in turn, pay rent to the corporation, so that a small sum of money has been required, once past the initial endowment, to maintain the apartment program. Patients are generally discharged in groups of from two to five, depending upon the size of the apartment. Since its inception in 1967, the program has grown to acquire a total of 13 apartments, in which 68 discharged chronically ill patients currently reside. A total of 182 discharged patients has been served by the apartment program to date. Occupancy rate in the apartments has been 87 percent. When a single vacancy occurs in an apartment (owing to death, rehospitalization, or—not at all infrequently—acceptance by a previously rejecting family of a patient who has now demonstrated ability to live in the community), the remaining residents participate in the selection of a replacement and have veto power over recommendations made by the staff.

A community housing resource which has been particularly useful for geriatric patients is a type of group residence which provides essentially hotel services—meals and minimal room housekeeping—with little additional supervision. These residences are licensed by the Department of Health of New York State, though the safety and staffing requirements are considerably less stringent than for nursing homes or chronic care hospitals. Great use of these residences is made by the Bronx State Hospital, particularly for the aged population whom the families in our communities will no longer care for. The initial experience was that discharging patients to such residences generally resulted in a very short stay in the community and early return to the hospital, because of the lack of services offered by these private, profit-making residences. Consequently, hospital staff are now deployed to provide social services, regular medical checkups, and organized group activities on the premises of the residence. The result has been a decided improvement in patient behavior and a much slower rate of return to hospital.

Halfway houses, foster homes, nursing homes, and, of course, return to the patient's own family, complete the range of residential resources we have available for housing chronically ill patients in the community. It is important to emphasize that any point along the continuum of autonomy and independence may come to represent a resting place for a chronically psychotic patient. To insist on an all-or-none division into hospital versus fully independent community life is simply unrealistic. This may appear to be a pessimistic note, implying a recognition that the chronically psychotic patient will never be totally "cured" and rendered capable of living like the rest of us. It is our view that this is our problem—the problem of the observers—rather than of the patients we are observing. It has been demonstrated that the presentation of a wooden facsimile of a monkey will terrify a colony of monkeys. In a related experiment, a fish trapped in a plastic bubble and released back into his school to swim his wobbly course will scatter the other fish in apparent terror. We suggest that much of the behavior of mental health professionals is like that of the monkeys and the fish. We cannot abide the wobbliness and woodenness among us, and our anxiety becomes translated into an urgent need to make the "deviants" just like ourselves. The victims of this therapeutic ambition to make all chronically psychotic patients "normal" are, of course, the patients. It is our conviction that if we make provision in the community for a range of wobbliness and woodenness, we will in the end, paradoxically, move further toward our present goal of "cure" than insistence upon polarizing humanity into the "sick" and the "well" will permit.

LIAISON PROGRAMS

Coequal in importance, in our experience, with the principle of graded adaptational opportunities for the community treatment of chronically psychotic patients is the principle of continuity of care. We mean by this the organization of mental health service delivery in such a manner that patients are cared for by a unified and cooperating group of mental health workers, whatever the modality and wherever the locus of treatment. It is remarkable that institutions—and there are many—can continue for years to refer patients to alternative treatment programs (e.g., from an inpatient ward to an outpatient clinic), fully aware that only 15 percent or fewer of the patients so referred make and keep an appointment. Our experience has been, for example, that the simple device of making a specific appointment, with a specific, named therapist increases this figure to over 50 percent, and the added step of having the clinic therapist or even his representative meet the patient on the wards prior to discharge, discuss the necessity for aftercare, and make a specific appointment increases initial attendance at the clinic to over 90 percent.

Given the administrative fragmentation of service agencies in the Bronx—under city, state, federal, and private auspices—territorial disputes are virtually assured, and the chronically psychotic patient, along with the aged, the addict, and the mentally retarded (and most particularly if the patient is black and poor) can be expected to be the target for exclusion from all. Conversely, the young, white, college-trained, articulate neurotic patient (and most particularly if she is attractive) often can find a number of agencies competing to provide her with treatment. This is perhaps not the appropriate occasion for a detailed sorting out of the many elements involved. The continued preeminence which the psychoanalytic model holds in American psychiatry, the racial and class biases, the reluctance of mental health professionals to risk failure in treating conditions which tend not to respond to current approaches when so many potentially responsive patients continue to be available—all these and other forces constitute the matrix within which the community-based treatment of the chronically psychotic patient must be carried out. Our concern has therefore, of necessity, been directed to insuring the establishment of liaison arrangements among the component elements in the mental health network so that continuity of care may be provided to chronically psychotic patients. A variety of patterns have emerged, four of which merit brief description. In each of these arrangements, the bickering between the inpatient and outpatient units about who is responsible for the patient has disappeared, and the rate of patients keeping initial clinic appointments after discharge has risen to 90 percent or more. Rehospitalization rates have begun to decline, although this trend is not yet statistically significant.

Liaison Between Hospital and Community Mental Health Center

Two community mental health centers are located in the Bronx, one of which we would suggest approximates a model liaison arrangement with a state mental hospital. The director of inpatient services of the Soundview–Throgs Neck Community Mental Health Center is responsible for the 50-bed unit operated by the center in the community, and he is also the chief of service for the 100-bed Soundview service at the Bronx State Hospital, which is responsible for patients in the same geographical area. He uses a single admitting room—in the community hospital—from which patients may be admitted to either unit. Generally, patients requiring longer hospitalization are admitted, or transferred, to the state mental hospital. The flexibility he enjoys can be illustrated by the following example. One of his wards at the state hospital is a hotel ward, and patients from the community hospital may, in preparation for discharge, be transferred to the state hospital if it is felt that the experience in minimally supervised living offered by the hotel ward would be useful. Case conferences are held which staff of both the community and state hospitals attend. The center operates three town clinics, one in each of the three demographically distinct communities which compose the center's catchment area, and each town clinic has a liaison staff which escorts patients into the hospital, maintains contact during hospitalization, and participates in discharge planning, including the specific scheduling of initial visits to the town clinic when the patient is ready to leave the hospital. Over 90 percent of these clinic appointments are kept. This liaison pattern between hospital and community mental health center is gradually being replicated in our relationship with the other such center in our hospital district, the Lincoln Hospital Community Mental Health Center.

Liaison Between Hospital and Comprehensive Health Center

A recent development in general health care, modeled to a degree after the community mental health center, is the health maintenance organization (HMO). This device, which is likely to be the central agency in a national health program, provides general medical, pediatric, and prenatal care on an ambulatory basis to population groups of from 20,000 to 40,000 in defined geographical areas. Like mental health centers, the HMOs attempt to develop health consciousness and to establish preventive as well as treatment programs. A further similarity is that in both extensive use is made of nonprofessional or paraprofessional health workers.

One of the units at the state mental hospital—the Crotona Park service—is a cluster of wards providing hospitalization for psychiatric patients from an area also served by the Martin Luther King Jr. Comprehensive Neighborhood Health Center, an HMO providing general medical, pediatric, dental, and prenatal care, but not psychiatric care, on an ambulatory basis to a population of about 45,000 persons, 90 percent of whom are black or Puerto Rican. Recently we have begun to discharge patients from the subarea served by the King center to the family care teams of that center, and to provide a psychiatric consultant to each family care team to attend the weekly meetings of the team. Our consultants serve as advisors on the psychiatric care, not only of the discharged chronically psychotic patients, but of all patients with emotional problems seen by the family care workers and the team professionals. An evaluation study of this program has just begun. Our impression is that this pattern of supervision of psychiatric aftercare treatment by a team providing comprehensive medical care is a more effective and far less costly approach to community care for chronically psychotic patients than either an after-care clinic or a mental hygiene clinic.

Liaison Between Mental Hospital and General Hospital Department of Psychiatry

The great bulk of the area for which our Crotona Park service is responsible, encompassing 140,000 persons as against the 45,000 served by the Martin Luther King Jr. Center, lies within the district of a general voluntary hospital, the Bronx-Lebanon Hospital. The department of psychiatry of this hospital is not mandated, nor does it have the resources, to provide outpatient aftercare services to patients discharged from the Bronx State Hospital. A quid pro quo was therefore effected whereby Bronx State Hospital pays the salaries of one psychiatrist and one social worker recruited by the director of psychiatry of the Bronx-Lebanon Hospital; in return, the mental hygiene clinic of the latter hospital provides aftercare treatment to patients discharged from our hospital. Parenthetically, our experience, contrary to that reported by others, is that the chronically psychotic patient does better when treated in a general psychiatric clinic than when segregated in a separate aftercare clinic; 38 percent of patients from that area treated in the state aftercare clinics were returned to the hospital in a year, as compared with 20 percent of patients treated at the Bronx-Lebanon mental hygiene clinic. More significant, 20 times as many patients continued in treatment after 2 years in the mental hygiene clinic as in the segregated aftercare clinic. The liaison pattern between Bronx State Hospital and Bronx-Lebanon Hospital has been replicated with the department of psychiatry of a municipal general hospital, the Lincoln Hospital, serving another area of the Bronx, with the additional feature of having permanent liaison mental health workers identified on each Lincoln Hospital service ward at Bronx State Hospital.

Liaison Between Hospital and Staffed Aftercare Clinic

One Bronx State Hospital service, the Williamsbridge-Fordham service, consists of a cluster of wards responsible for the psychiatric hospitalization of patients from a geographical area served by a municipal hospital which accepts chronically psychotic patients into its mental hygiene clinic only in very limited numbers. This service, after a trial of a geographically distant state aftercare clinic which proved highly unsatisfactory, organized its own outpatient department, using professional and nonprofessional staff members from the wards as clinic therapists, rather than a separate, discontinuous clinic staff. Some patients, deeply involved in group therapy on the ward at the time of discharge, may have their outpatient appointments initially made to the wards to coincide with the group meetings. The results have been salutary; the rehospitalization rate has dropped from 51 percent to 33 percent and is still declining, and the retention rate in treatment after 2 years rose from close to zero in the state clinic to about 50 percent. The Williamsbridge-Fordham service outpatient clinic is located on the grounds of the mental hospital, though some distance from the wards of that service. Ideally, the service would like to locate its outpatient department entirely off the hospital grounds and in the community to emphasize for patients their changed status, but it plans to retain the practice of using the same treatment staff for inpatient and outpatient phases of treatment. Three other Bronx State Hospital services—the Riverdale-North Central, the Bronx Municipal, and the Highbridge services—operate their own aftercare clinics, the last with a separate clinic staff, and the other two with shared ward and clinic responsibilities by the service staff.

SUMMARY

We have attempted to describe a 1000-bed multimodality, community-oriented state mental hospital which serves as a hub for a regional network of community mental health programs for a population of 1.5 million. It is our conviction that this is a viable, and perhaps the most desirable, model for the delivery of mental health services to a region. It avoids the risk of converting the hospital, again, into a custodial repository for "untreatable" patients rejected by community facilities; it provides flexibility and a range of choices for selecting a treatment facility for a given patient; it provides a spectrum of treatment approaches; it maximizes the loci of precare and aftercare modalities by sharing the resources of the hospital and the community-based facilities; and it offers the possibility of effecting the fullest continuity of care to patients. Certainly, advances can be expected in pharmacological, milieu, family, group, and individual therapeutic approaches in the period immediately ahead, and these advances may change dramatically the problem of the care and treatment of chronically psychotic patients. In the meantime, the twin goals we urge upon any mental health service delivery system are (1) a full range of both hospital and community treatment, rehabilitative, residential, social, and recreational facilities to accommodate the full range of abilities and disabilities of these patients; and (2) liaison arrangements among all treatment resources, to provide optimally for the continuity of patient care.

REFERENCES

1. Solomon, H: The American Psychiatric Association in relation to American psychiatry. Am. J. Psychiatry 115:1, 1958
2. Caplan RB: Psychiatry and the Community in Nineteenth-Century America. New York, Basic Books, 1969
3. Glasscote R, Sussex J, Cumming, E, Smith L: The Community Mental Health Center: An Interim Appraisal. Washington, DC,

Joint Information Service of the American Psychiatric Association and the National Association for Mental Health, 1969
4. May P: Treatment of Schizophrenia. New York, Science House, 1968
5. Grinspoon L, Ewalt J, Shader R: Psychotherapy and pharmacotherapy in chronic schizophrenia Am J Psychiatry 124:67–74, 1968

William Goldman, M.D.

2

Two Models for Organizing Mental Health Care Delivery

Large segments of our population exhibit deep anxieties and frustrations when asked about the availability of good health care, according to an in-depth national survey conducted for the Blue Cross Association as long ago as December 1968. Two thirds of the general public feel that you can't get a doctor in an emergency; 40 percent of the general public (and two thirds of the poor) worry that they will be unable to pay a doctor if they can locate one; and more than half the general public (and two thirds of the poor) told interviewers they were terrified of a serious illness that would disable the breadwinner and wipe out all family savings. Although not specifically addressing mental health care, the above findings are central to much of the increasing investigation of new methods of delivering human services.

A great deal has been written about the consortium model which has become increasingly popular with the expansion of community mental health centers. Two prominent examples are the San Francisco Westside Community Mental Health Center, Inc.,[1-5] and the West Philadelphia Community Mental Health Consortium.[6-8] I should like to summarize briefly the Westside center model and then compare and contrast it with the Bronx program described in Chapter 1. I will attempt to raise some generic issues regarding organizational structures and dynamics essential to delivery of mental health services and establishment of a system of mental health care.

THE WESTSIDE CENTER

The Westside Community Mental Health Center, Inc., of San Francisco opened its doors to bring its services to the total population of the Westside district of San Francisco on January 1, 1969. This followed a 2-year period of planning

31

and community organization aimed at achieving comprehensive mental health services, not by duplicating or replacing existing services, but rather by coordinating and improving existing programs and filling in the gaps. To achieve this objective, various Westside mental health agencies, which had historically operated autonomously, formed an organization to integrate their services and thereby provide a new mechanism for the prevention and treatment of emotional problems of Westside residents.

In October 1966, the first letter of invitation was sent to some of the major Westside mental health agencies from the department of psychiatry at Mt. Zion Hospital. By mid-1967, nine heterogeneous agencies—Jewish Family Service and Family Service of San Francisco; a halfway house, Conard House; Suicide Prevention, Inc.; California Medical Clinic for Psychotherapy; and four psychiatric departments of general hospitals—committed themselves to form a new partnership. Because the majority of San Francisco's mental health facilities were located in the Westside district, it was clear from the onset that there would be little purpose in a program of building construction. The challenge was to make maximal use of existing facilities and to concentrate on gaps in services which had to be met outside the Westside area or not at all. Amendment of Public Law 88-164 at the federal level (allowing for staffing grants), a more liberal formula for state reimbursement of local community programs, and a new emphasis on regional health planning made this a most propitious time for collaborative efforts.

In conjunction with representatives of the community mental health services of the city and county of San Francisco, the California Department of Mental Hygiene, and representatives from the regional office of the National Institute of Mental Health, planning proceeded to submit a community mental health center staffing grant. The Westside consortium therefore represented a coalition of independent private, nonprofit agencies banded together in a new way toward carrying out a major public program with major public financing. The forging of a new alliance between the private and public sector was possible in San Francisco, since the city had already taken the lead in California in developing contractual services with individual private mental health agencies.

In reviewing the first year of the Westside center's development, we saw a rather complex series of processes occurring simultaneously at various levels. It must be borne in mind that these processes varied considerably, both with the individuals and with the agencies involved. Regarding participation in the Westside center, these processes included, in rough chronological order, (1) education, (2) reassurance about aims and objectives, (3) wide involvement of key people holding responsible positions in the mental health agencies and programs, (4) the evolution of the individuals involved into a group with the setting of preliminary goals and working through of long-standing doubts, (5) the gradual transformation of suspicion into trust, of unfamiliarity and ignorance into awareness and acceptance, (6) the clarification of potential gratifications in continued or further involvement in the center, (7) the growth of cooperative planning and sharing of program aspirations, (8) a shift from agency to center considerations, and (9) the beginning of identification with the concepts and objectives of the center.

We accepted the premise that health care was a right and not a privilege, a concept that inevitably led to a new view of community participation in planning and programming for health care delivery. Today, community participation in this process is often talked about in terms of consumer participation. There have always been consumers in positions of power on boards of hospitals and health care agencies. The term "consumer," as used today, is a euphemism for the poor. In the decade of the 1960s, it usually meant blacks, though it included in the East, Puerto Ricans, in the West, Chicanos, and more recently in the Bay Area, Asians and native Americans.

The Westside center began with 9 agencies and has now grown to 19. These agencies historically developed in what is now known as the Westside catchment area, a heterogeneous district composed of an upper-class section, a range of middle-class and working-class white areas, as well as a black ghetto, Japantown, and the hippie community of Haight-Ashbury.

The first organizational stage in the development of the Westside center focused on getting these independent and sometimes rivalrous agencies to begin to work together toward coordinating services. This stage took approximately a year. The second stage, which took somewhat less of the following year, was that of getting the nonagency community involved and identified with the Westside center before it opened its doors. Once we were assured that the Westside center could become a reality and that funding would be made available for it on the federal and state level, we began to contact all the diverse groups we could learn about, and eventually these numbered approximately 85.

Our plan was to seek the support of these groups in acquiring the necessary local matching funds from the city, encourage them to attend the first community forum at which the community advisory board was to be elected, and maintain their ongoing involvement in the operations of the Westside center. We did not have a long-range plan. Our schedule was only to open our doors with the essential services necessary to make the Westside center eligible for funding so that all residents of the Westside could receive care in their own community and would no longer have to go to the county hospital. Future planning and development were to be under the direction of the new alliance among professionals, agency representatives, and the community. The community was dubious, at best, but willing to help and to go along for awhile to see if we would live up to our promises.

The first Westside community mental health forum, in September 1968, was a successful experiment in democracy. The forum nominated and unanimously elected representatives to constitute the community advisory board. These members, combined with the agency representatives on the board of directors, constituted an excellent cross section of the total community. The first task of this interim community advisory board was to elect one half of the board of directors of the center (the other one half consisted of the representatives of the component agencies), and to do this before services began January 1, 1969. The board of directors of the center is the policy-making body and fiscal agent for all Westside programs. There were two other charges to the interim community advisory board: Within nine months, it was to create the bylaws for the permanent community advisory board and to convene the second forum by June 1969 to elect the permanent board. These charges were accomplished on schedule.

After the first months of testing, the community representatives clearly established their leadership of the board and formulated their priorities. The first priority was the inclusion of youth at the top level of direction of the center, i.e., the board of directors. The second priority was the inclusion of indigenous self-help programs for drug users as full members of the consortium once they incorporated and received their tax-free status. The third was the development of a comprehensive drug-treatment program with particular emphasis on narcotics addiction. Within a short period, a drug council had come into being, staffed by the central office with representatives of all the programs interested in caring for persons with these problems, and preparation of a new grant for a comprehensive program was under way. The fourth concern was for children's services, with special focus on day care for sick children of working mothers and care of neglected and dependent children traditionally housed at the grossly inadequate youth guidance center.

The community advisory board, impatient and committed, took the initiative from the board of directors in pushing active community support and involvement in the programmatic, fiscal, and personnel operations of the center.

In this pluralistic system with a heterogeneity of agencies, disciplines, fiscal arrangements, schools of thought and style, another organizational task was the creation of new intrasystem alliances among the mental health professionals. Major effort was expended to break down the barrier to treatment that had traditionally existed through each agency's idiosyncratic eligibility procedures. The Westside community had never had 24-hour emergency service, day treatment center, organized consultation and education service, or inpatient services for public patients. There did exist extensive outpatient services throughout the consortium and three small private inpatient units at Mt. Zion, Pacific Presbyterian, and St. Mary's. These institutions made a major commitment to the program by allocating over 50 percent of their inpatient beds to the new Westside community program. It was agreed that the most logical place to house the new 24-hour walk-in psychiatric emergency service was Mt. Zion, which was most centrally located and accessible and could best staff this kind of program. The major breakthrough came in the agreement from the three inpatient units that all patients to be admitted would be funneled first through this single emergency service or at least cleared through it without duplicate evaluation for hospitalization. This radical change in admission procedures was also applied to the new day treatment center at Pacific Presbyterian. Each patient referred from one of the consortium agencies would have to be accepted in the program. A commitment was also made by the consortium agencies to shift their existing priorities for services in their preexisting programs so that Westside residents received first priority for care regardless of whether there was a new contract for a new service.

Much of this was achieved by significant shifts in philosophy in the consortium agencies toward reduction in length of hospital stay, emphasis on alternatives to hospitalization, crisis intervention, home visiting, and aftercare. This change allowed the program to absorb the greatly increased volume of patients for treatment and evaluation, both voluntary and involuntary, necessitated by changes in the law during 1969 as well as by the newly available and accessible community programs.

Another factor that had concerned the center from the outset was reaching the underserved poor and minority group population in our catchment area. The black population of the Westside is approximately 30 percent of the total population, yet none of the preexisting outpatient services had more than 10–15 percent black patients in their service load. By the end of the first year of Westside center operations, the outpatient programs had increased services to black patients by 5–10 percent, the day treatment and inpatient services were approaching the one third mark; and the emergency, crisis-intervention, and home visiting services had already surpassed that. By the third year of operation, the black population in our treatment services was proportionate to that in the general population of our catchment area.

The financial organization of the Westside was based on the concept that no new superagency was to be developed, and that the central office would be responsible only for coordinating and evaluating programs and would not perform any direct services. The central office, acting on behalf of the board as fiscal agent, serves in the capacity of fiscal intermediary between government funding sources and the agencies with which there are subcontracts for all new and old direct Westside services.

This arrangement provided fiscal flexibility, with acceptance of the fact that costs could vary in different agencies for the same service. It also recognized that these established agencies, many of which were recognized vendors for the California medicaid program (Medi-Cal), could in turn bill all third-party payers for eligible patients before billing the Westside center itself. In fact, it was stipulated in all the contracts that the agencies were required to do so. This arrangement also made the most of the contacts these agencies had for bringing in additional philanthropic aid and Community Chest funds to assist in the initiation of new programs. In addition, it tapped into the existing procedures for collecting direct patient fees most appropriately and completely.

In order to assist the center in achieving its primary goal of responsible patient management, a computerized human accountability system was established. This system has three main functions: (1) to maintain a centralized record of all transactions of patients with all component facilities of the center, (2) to provide a series of messages to participating facilities alerting them to patient needs for collaboration or other attention, and (3) to make periodic statistical analyses of the entire psychiatric care delivery system for purposes of program monitoring.

A derivative, the Westside management information system (MIS), is designed to synthesize that information which describes the present operation of the Westside system and to allow the management to perform individual program monitoring and program evaluation. In a general sense, it serves as part of the substantive information for program planning and in the future could serve as a fundamental system for an overall project evaluation of Westside.

The operation of the system is intended to minimize the peripheral work surrounding direct services (i.e., paperwork) and at the same time gather sufficient information to completely characterize the agencies' operations. The projected uses of the MIS are further extended from the simple recording of patient-therapist interactions and bed counts of inpatient facilities to include budget analysis, patient billing, cost effectiveness analyses, a personal information system, a follow-up system, and a standard statistical information system (i.e., census and other data). This information will provide Westside with a capability that it has not had in the past and that few mental health centers now have—the capacity to provide effective and meaningful feedback to agencies regarding their performance.

In the new Westside MIS, only two forms are required by the system for patient management:

1. An intake interview which is completed only once, upon entry into the Westside system through any Westside operating agency, and which from then on is updated but never repeated.
2. A transaction encounter report, which is a record of each therapist's patient contacts and of each patient's status change. The transaction encounter report is completed by each therapist or inpatient unit officer each day and is transmitted to the Westside central office daily.

The MIS reduces the paper flow by eliminating five forms required on each patient and provides the information required by the funding sources.

The kind of responsive and flexible program growth that has been possible over the past 5-year period of Westside center operations illustrates the potential that exists in the mental health field today. Not only have additional existing agencies joined the consortium, but new grass-roots agencies were brought into being under the aegis of the consortium. A comprehensive aftercare and rehabilitative service for chronically ill patients was developed simultaneously with preventive programs emphasizing family-oriented services to children and youth. Replicas of the Westside center system have been attempted in a number of communities across the country. This is in addition to the explicit move toward this model by the other San Francisco community mental health centers. The maximizing of a long-term, stable, multiple-source funding base is also evident in this approach, as is its potential for the entire physical and social health field.

Additional facets of the Westside program will be mentioned in the following comparison with the Bronx program. I will attempt to highlight and reemphasize certain issues raised by Dr. Zwerling as well as to contrast certain alternate pathways developed by these two different programs in attempting to meet common goals.

WESTSIDE AND THE BRONX: A COMPARISON

Dr. Zwerling's discussion provides a succinct historical synopsis of contemporary trends in the field of community mental health. It is worth noting, however, that his description is a view of a process, of an end point in the development of quality mental health service delivery systems in this country. The current experience of ongoing experimentation and refinement in system building reminds us continually of the need to explore and leave open all options while recognizing current realistic limitations in the state of our knowledge. Simultaneously maintaining the momentum and enthusiasm of the community mental health movement requires the encouragement and nurturance of the entire mental health field as new generations confront age-old dilemmas as well as the frustrations of professional ignorance and helplessness in altering social patterns and structures.

The increasing participation of the citizenry in policy making for community mental health programs is proportionate to the growing level of awareness and acceptance of the broad psychosocial issues facing the field and thereby necessarily involving the general public. The sophisticated interest and criticism by the media and by consumer interest groups (e.g., the Nader report from the Center for the Study of Responsive Law[9]) challenge one of our commitments in community mental health. They test our willingness to welcome all concerned parties into our professional sanctum sanctorum, to open our program-planning and decision-making processes to scrutiny by all, to share the power associated with these functions, and to replace the mysticism surrounding our professional activities by the most open and rational processes available.

Like the Nader report, an example of investigative journalism in our field, Dr. Zwerling raises in Chapter 1 the caveat that community mental health centers, as some have operated to date, may contribute to the very thing they were intended to reduce—chronicity. Yet it is possible to see already that other appropriately structured community-based programs have been able to avoid the pitfall of "skimming" (devoting the majority of therapeutic attention to the least disordered persons). Skimming is often associated with the absence of appropriate ongoing linkages with the previous state hospital repositories of the most mentally disabled. It perpetuates the isolation of one segment of the population from community rehabilitative services. The obligation for forging programmatic partnerships remains equally on the shoulders of the old and the new treatment systems, with much more than superficial attention paid to the basic principle of continuity of care.

One of the difficulties discussed by Dr. Zwerling is usually clustered under the heading of "dumping" (extrusion of difficult, socially rejected, or unmanageable patients). One way to minimize dumping might be to alter the fiscal underpinning of the total mental health care system he describes. This can be achieved to a significant degree by the creation of a unified fiscal system with a single budget allocation from a specific government source (a method that currently applies best to state funding of mental health programs). Such a system would finally allow "the dollar to follow the patients." Although not a panacea, I know of no other single basic structural change that can so readily provide the flexibility needed to rapidly adapt programs to clients needs. Similarly, it ensures the forging of the necessary alliances of all the vested interests in the total mental health care system if for no other reason than to survive. This single step would go far to assure the growth of true *systems* of care.

Many in the field remain convinced that even the best application of the above principles can still only reduce, not eliminate, the number of failures within our treatment systems. We cannot yet see an end to that group of clients who will be filtered out from even the most complete and highest quality comprehensive system. These persons may require indefinite open-ended, ongoing protective care and shelter. The perspective of the community mental health movement is only one part of the evolutionary process of achieving optimum care for disturbed persons.

The model elucidated by Dr. Zwerling of the state hospital as a central service linkage factor is clearly a reasonable one which should be closely examined, especially in communities where the historical development of mental health services predisposes to the adoption or modification of this particular concept—a university-affiliated hospital not too distant from the population to be served.

The question should be asked whether state hospitals should continue to be conceived of as treatment centers for chronically ill patients only. There is already ample evidence that early-intervention, community-based acute treatment programs are not always best equipped to treat all the individuals who come to or are brought to them. It is highly questionable whether large amounts of money should be expended to duplicate expensive specialized facilities for a small number of clients who could be well treated as acutely ill patients in accessible *nearby* state hospitals given the appropriate program development. This concept is based, of course, on adequate provisions for continuity of care, such as continuity of therapeutic personnel, which would link the state hospitals with the community-based programs. (The need is still present for a protected and, if necessary, locked facility for brief intense treatment lasting days or weeks.) This need should be increasingly rare when appropriate community alternatives have been developed. I am not at all sure that it is necessary or even appropriate to duplicate these highly specialized facilities in every community, for surely some will be too small to have effective programs. It may be far more sensible for such a specialized facility to be shared by neighboring communities. In certain locales this function could be best offered by a nearby state hospital.

Program planners should also note that there is ample evidence to suggest certain predictable patterns and trends in the first few years after the establishment of new community programs. Exaggerated promises have been made, either implicitly or occasionally explicitly, that the use of 24-hour care would be reduced dramatically soon after the onset of new comprehensive programs. In fact, quite the opposite has been shown to be the case. The creation of new accessible, available, and relevant neighborhood services will lead to a utilization peak for acute and intensive services lasting from 1 to 2 years. Consistently, many persons who previously avoided either distant or stigmatized mental health services (such as state hospitals) begin to make long overdue use of local facilities and programs. This phenomenon must not only be planned for, it must be budgeted for! It is characteristically American that newness is sought after regardless of content, quality, or proven value.

In the program I am most familiar with, at the Westside center in San Francisco, after over 2 years of planning and data gathering, we decided to set up our new programs and staff them with the expectation that there would be a 100 percent increase in utilization of our new local services over those previously available at the county hospital and state hospitals. Within 6 months after beginning operations, the utilization rates in our services were already four times greater than the baseline rates present before we opened our doors.

I would like to emphasize here the need for great caution. In light of the many economic and social factors beyond our control that continually impinge on the growth and development of the population at large, we are hard put to predict the kind of rate of manifestation of problems which may come to our attention. We should bear in mind, therefore, the critical need for a pluralistic approach to program development. The essence of community mental health should dictate that no national or international template can be imposed across all communities. At best, a variety of demonstrably useful models should be offered which can be modified appropriately to the uniqueness of each community. Simultaneously, the development of new programmatic variations and concepts must be encouraged. This ongoing process must be interwoven throughout the entire community mental health movement. If ever there was a human service system that should tolerate built-in change and adaptation to change, mental health care is the one.

The history, mores, and resources of each community, rather than new preconceived models, must be the basis upon which any meaningful service system can be built. These factors are the critical determinants of the options and the possibilities for future development.

The body of Dr. Zwerling's chapter concerns itself with the treatment concepts of his program. The breadth and versatility of his approach deserves imitation. One salient feature of program development that emerges from his description is the way programs are predetermined by the physical structures they arise from and to which they are often chained. The contrast with our experience in San Francisco is striking. Several years ago, the decision was made to move entirely out of the antiquated county hospital. Following or preceding acute hospitalization in local general hospital inpatient units, the five San Francisco community mental health centers developed a diverse, flexible, and ofttimes innovative spectrum of residential alternatives to hospital care. No construction was involved. The services utilized renovated residential property scattered throughout the city. They range from 24-hour professionally supervised emergency housing available for days or weeks if necessary, through a spectrum of halfway-house facilities linked to outpatient rehabilitation programs and day treatment centers. Many clients spend up to 12 months in various facilities depending on their need. Other residential programs accommodate clients without a time limit. Linked to this system is a series of apartments for supervised group living as further non-time-limited transitional facilities. As their experience increases, these programs are able to accept more and more acutely disturbed persons, often obviating the need for hospitalization or rehospitalization. Sensitivity to differing ethnic and cultural life styles necessitated a range of options within the above-mentioned programs for the various subgroups of the population.

It is important to stress that the clients usually do not remain in these facilities during the day, but are in some form of outpatient therapeutic program while pursuing schooling, vocations, and avocations. A strong emphasis on vocational rehabilitation permeates this program, and this includes acceptance as goals for such rehabilitation many alternatives to full-time employment.

The common problem of discontinuity of care in the prevalent fragmented nonsystem of mental health services in urban areas is appropriately emphasized by Dr. Zwerling in his explication of the various liaison functions performed within the network he describes. The development of an automated methodology for tracking clients in such complex systems is still in an experimental phase in a number of such centers, including the Westside in San Francisco.[10-12] One facet of activity in this area in Dr. Zwerling's program is the use of the new mental health professional to perform some of these functions. It should be pointed out that the substitution of the new careerist or so-called paraprofessional can be and is often perceived by poor and minority groups as another form of second-class treatment and institutional racism. A better approach involves vigorous recruitment and training of minority mental health professionals serving nonwhite clients.

Dr. Zwerling's model clearly represents the application of the principle of maximum utilization of existing resources. This is a critical determinant of the future viability and stability of evolving systems of mental health care delivery. It is also in full accord with the American accretive tradition of human services development. The Bronx program represents the kind of institutional dynamism all too frequently lacking in systems antedating the community mental health movement. On the other hand, contemporary products of this movement are by no means immune to the institutional ossification all too familiar on the American health scene.

REFERENCES

1. Bolman WM: The mental health consortium. In Bellak L, Barten HH (eds): Progress in Community Mental Health, vol II, New York, Grune & Stratton, 1972
2. Bolman WM: Community control of the community mental health center: II. Case examples. Am J Psychiatry 129:181–186, 1972
3. Bolman WM, Goldman W: San Francisco Westside Community Mental Health Center, Inc.: Development of a mental health consortium of private agencies. In Levenson A, Beigel A (eds): The Community Mental Health Center: Strategies and Programs, New York, Basic Books, 1972
4. Martens H, Warren C: The multi-agency community mental health center: Administrative and organizational relationships. Report submitted to the NIMH by the National Academy of Public Administration, Washington, DC, 1971, Appendix E and I
5. Gattozzi A: San Francisco's Westside: A community mental health center serves the people. In Segal J (ed): NIMH Mental Health Program, Reports-5. Rockville, Md, National Institute of Mental Health, 1972, pp 174–187
6. Leopold RL: The West Philadelphia mental health consortium: Administrative planning in a multi-hospital catchment area. Am J Psychiatry 124:69–76, 1967
7. Leopold RL: Urban problems and the community mental health center: Multiple mandates, difficult choices. I. The West

Philadelphia community mental health consortium: Background and current status. Panel discussion at the 47th Annual Meeting of the American Psychiatric Association, San Francisco, Mar 23–24, 1970

8. Leopold RL: Partnership for mental health: Complexities in a community mental health center. I. The consortium concept. Panel discussion at the 22nd Institute on Hospital and Community Psychiatry, Philadelphia, Sept 21–24, 1970

9. Chu F, Trotter S: The Mental Health Complex. Part I. Community Mental Health Center. Washington, DC Center for Study of Responsive Law, 1972

10. Kiresuk TJ, Sherman RE: Goal attainment scaling: A general method for evaluating community mental health programs. Community Ment Health J 4: 443–453, 1968

11. Elpers JR: Management information system: Tools for integrating human services. Paper presented at the 24th Institute on Hospital and Community Psychiatry, St. Louis, Sept 1972

12. Bloom B: Human accountability in a community mental health center: Report of an automated system. Community Ment Health J 4:251–260, 1972

Harvey H. Barten, M.D.

3

A Suburban Clinic in Transition

This chapter describes the evolution of a suburban community mental health clinic whose budget has grown fourfold in as many years, even without the stimulus of federal funding under the Community Mental Health Centers Act. The multifaceted program which has developed typifies the prospects and problems of many free-standing clinics; throughout the country they are seeking practical ways of reshaping organization and objectives to meet the challenge of community mental health in the economically uncertain 1970s. The latter part of this paper discusses some broader issues which affect community clinics.

The Guidance Center of New Rochelle, the largest outpatient psychiatric clinic in Westchester County, is one of more than 1100 free-standing community psychiatric clinics in the United States.[1] Typically, it was begun with limited objectives; its widening scope of activities in recent years could hardly have been foreseen when it opened its doors in 1942 as the first privately financed child-guidance clinic in Westchester County. Its name, increasingly inaccurate, has somehow stuck.

A broadening of the original intent first occurred in 1945, at the close of World War II, when the guidance center became one of the first clinics in Westchester to establish a veterans' rehabilitation division. It was not until 1958 that the contract with Westchester County was expanded to support the development of a full-scale adult clinic.

In the mid-1960s, a reinvigorated community mental health movement began to influence American psychiatrists to undertake more ambitious and comprehensive community projects. Responding to emerging concepts and opportunities, the Guidance Center accelerated the pace of developing multifaceted services. New approaches were sought for growing problems such as drug addiction, as well as for long-standing needs such as those of previously underserved patients with chronic psychoses.

The introduction of new therapeutic strategies, the reexamination and retooling of existing programs, and the development of new concepts reflecting a public health model are transforming the clinic into a comprehensive community mental health center. As we become conversant with the total mental health needs in the community, we are developing a wide range of services to meet those needs. This has required a redefining of the objectives of psychotherapy so that limited resources can be deployed to the best advantage of the total community. We have had to decide which of myriad needs would receive priority status, which must await future attention, and which can be handled by other community resources. The clinic staff has moved into the community, both to do active case finding and to collaborate with human service resources such as the educational, welfare, employment, and judicial systems. The development of a network of coordination is fundamental to the community mental health center concept: comprehensive, integrated helping services with increasing consumer participation in their design and execution.

Harsh economic realities have threatened the viability of community mental health innovations from their very beginnings. Free-standing clinics like ours have been particularly vulnerable. Clinics affiliated with general hospitals are more likely to have their inevitable deficits underwritten by the more solid underpinnings of their self-supporting inpatient services.

SOME VITAL STATISTICS

The Guidance Center of New Rochelle is the major mental health resource for a catchment area of about 135,000 people in a portion of southern Westchester County (also including Larchmont, Mamaroneck, and Pelham) where pockets of severe poverty abut areas of declining affluence. About 15 percent of the district's population is black, the greatest portion of whom are socioeconomically deprived. Over one third of the residents are of Italian extraction, mostly blue-collar workers. Since the clinic limits services primarily to those least able to afford them, over 50 percent of the patients it serves have family incomes of under $5000 per year and over half of these receive welfare assistance. Some 30 percent are black.

Presently the clinic occupies a three-story brick building centrally located in the business district of New Rochelle, within walking distance of bus and rail centers. The central office building houses facilities for a therapeutic nursery school, a day hospital, and a rehabilitation program for psychotic patients, in addition to offices for individual and group therapy provided for children and adults. Two satellite clinics also provide general mental health services. One is located in a black ghetto area in New Rochelle; the other is in Mamaroneck, at the northern end of the catchment area. The Guidance Center also operates two methadone maintenance clinics, located in commercial buildings in different parts of New Rochelle.

Funds for the operation of the Guidance Center are raised by a private board of directors, and are matched on a 50-50 basis by the New York State Department of Mental Hygiene, through a contract with the Westchester Community Mental Health Board. Initially, Westchester County provided additional seed money on a diminishing basis for developing adult services, but these funds have been exhausted. Special services, such as the methadone programs and the rehabilitation program, have been totally funded by the New York State Department of Mental Hygiene. The total operating budget now exceeds $1 million per year.

An average of over 80 applications is received each month, and about 1500 individuals receive direct services each year. Monthly clinic visits average 2000, not including the methadone clinics. Since the demand for services has increased by 5–6 percent each year, there has of necessity been a gradual shift to the greater utilization of short-term and group techniques. These programs have assumed critical importance and are described further below. Of equal importance, an effective community mental health program must allocate an increasing amount of time to consultation for numerous care givers in the community.

To complete the picture, the clinic maintains training programs for social work students, psychology interns, pastoral counseling students, psychiatric residents, paraprofessionals, and volunteers.

A SUBURBAN REFERRAL AND CONSULTATION NETWORK

A public health orientation[2] demands that a clinic extend its services to more than those sufficiently well motivated to want help and sufficiently well organized to find it. We have developed a network of formal and informal relationships with both care givers and key members of the community to find those with the greatest need, who otherwise might not seek treatment. It is through these contacts that we can get to the adaptive casualties who exist at varying degrees of visibility within the community: addicts, nonfunctioning psychotics, welfare mothers who function at a level far below their potential, and individuals in crisis who, without well-timed assistance, can become emotionally disabled.

A suburban setting permits the development of informal consultative relationships. In the more impersonal bureaucracy of the central city, agencies can be so inundated that they abandon all thought of operating on the level of personal contacts. Therapists in central-city mental health clinics can feel hopelessly frustrated by the formidable maze of overlapping agencies which they must work with or around. In suburban settings, it is far easier to develop mutually helpful relationships with agency workers who serve the same district and who are able to take a more personal interest in their clients. For example, our staff knows many of the social workers at the department of welfare, who freely and informally consult us about problem cases. We provide evaluation and treatment of their clients with a minimum of formality; they provide invaluable assistance in helping our patients to obtain welfare or medicaid assistance without customary delays or administrative runarounds.

In addition to the helping agents mentioned above, we have offered workshops to public health nurses, probation workers, child-protective services, community action programs, workers in street drug programs, and clergymen. We try to help them provide counseling to clients who have psychological problems. Reflecting the philosophy of community mental health,[3-5] we are helping care givers to assume more therapeutic roles when their clients bring them relatively uncomplicated problems; they learn to refer only clients with more complex needs to the more experienced therapists or special services in our clinic. In some instances we have worked with care givers who already possess impressive counseling abilities reflecting innate talents, accumulated experience, or both. Many of them tend to underrate these competencies and to look to mental health professionals as the only legitimate counseling agents. Sometimes our job is to help other care givers to credit their own capacities. They may need us more to sanction a broadening of their roles than to teach them new techniques. When necessary, we have provided weekly supervision: for example, helping a new street worker in a youthful drug-abuse program to expand his skills in counseling adolescent drug experimenters.

HANDLING THE PSYCHIATRIC POPULATION EXPLOSION

Fostering and enhancing counseling skills of other helping agents in the community keep referrals from inundating the clinic. Nevertheless, a successful program generates increasing numbers of applications which require a triage system to prevent lengthy delays. We are unwilling to tolerate waiting lists, an antitherapeutic way of handling, or discouraging, excessive numbers of applicants. Waiting lists multiply the dropout rate and squander the opportunity to provide therapeutic intervention at the critical moment when it may be most effective.[6] Selection for psychotherapy should not be on the basis of capacity to tolerate administrative obstacles and endless delays.

Our simplified intake system permits any individual who desires an appointment to apply directly and with minimum formality. When there is an emergency, the patient is seen at once; otherwise he receives an appointment for an interview within the next few days. Few patients are kept waiting more than 1 week. The first appointment is a screening evaluation with an experienced clinician who can quickly assess the severity of the current problem and establish an initial diagnostic impression. A sufficiently accurate working diagnosis can be established in over 90 percent of these rapid evaluations. Those who need treatment are then assigned to the most appropriate therapy program.

APPORTIONING LIMITED RESOURCES

Of the patients for whom we recommend psychotherapy in our clinic, about one third receive short-term individual or family counseling. If not actually in the midst of crisis situations, initial or recurrent, these patients generally manifest neurotic or familial difficulties which do not pervade all aspects of their lives.

Brief techniques are also employed for patients with complex problems when lengthier therapies are unacceptable, unavailable, or unlikely to be more effective.

Another third of the patients are referred to an appropriate group. Many of these patients have interpersonal or character problems, and some have received individual therapy in the past. Patients are more likely to be selected for group therapy if they already have some awareness of their problems and some motivation to get help, and are able to tolerate the initial stress of a group situation.

The remaining patients accepted for therapy are referred for programs which are open-ended in duration. Some have compounded or insidious problems for which brief therapies appear unsuitable. These include borderline schizophrenic patients who require long-term therapeutic relationships, patients with severe acting-out disorders, patients with alcohol and other addiction problems, and patients with long-standing, mixed neurotic disorders, such as panphobic housewives. Lengthier therapy is also considered for unmarried mothers living on welfare; many come from broken homes and have never been able to achieve a satisfactory life adjustment. Individuals such as these need help in sorting out and better coping with many problem areas of their lives; longer therapeutic relationships are likely to be more productive, when patients will accept them. Longer therapy is generally reserved for the more disturbed patients, not the "good treatment cases."[7-9] Naturally, we are as flexible in renegotiating the therapy contract for these patients as we are with short-term patients, when our initial therapeutic goals prove untenable. Psychotic patients who require multiphasic services are referred to our day hospital or rehabilitation program.

Since we instituted this system of immediate screening, we have reduced the percentage of unkept initial appointments from over 30 to under 10 percent. Patients who fail to keep initial appointments are recontacted by telephone; if their problem statement suggests serious difficulties, home visits are also employed, in an effort to get them to come to the clinic.

Not all those evaluated are accepted for psychotherapy. In some cases, a single session is sufficient to help an individual understand the nature of his problem, suggest alternative courses of action, or support positive steps he already may have taken to resolve the problem.[10] Other patients are advised to return to the referring agency for further help. We provide a report to the agency and, whenever possible, discuss diagnostic impressions and recommendations with a member of the agency staff. Some patients are referred to more appropriate therapeutic resources such as addiction programs directed by ex-addicts, Alcoholics Anonymous, vocational rehabilitation, or employment counseling.

SHORT-TERM PSYCHOTHERAPY

A range of brief therapeutic strategies is indispensable in enabling the clinic to provide immediate treatment to many patients with acute, recurring, and in some cases long-standing problems. Even therapists with more traditional orientations are becoming favorably impressed by the compelling advantages of short-term approaches, which I have discussed in detail elsewhere.[11-14] Particularly when previous coping patterns have been adequate, patients in crisis are obvious candidates. On the other hand, patients with chronic or recurring problems often will not accept help except during periods of acute distress. There will never be enough therapeutic resources to meet the needs of all who might benefit, and many patients will achieve only limited gains from treatment, no matter how long its duration. In some instances, brief therapy is the treatment of choice, restoring adaptive balance while avoiding regression or the induction of dependent attitudes which patients later may find difficult to relinquish. Our expanding spectrum of brief therapies includes conjoint therapies, family therapies, behaviorally oriented therapies, drug therapies, time-limited groups, and brief contact therapy.[11]

Brief therapy is an essential component of our treatment programs, but we feel no need to oversell it as the universal treatment of choice. Longer-term group and individual therapies are provided to individuals who should have them, particularly within the framework of our rehabilitation program. Longer-term patients are periodically reviewed to assure that their continuation in the clinic reflects persisting needs rather than habit.

Workshops in short-term therapy examine basic concepts and extrapolate from the growing experience within this field. We have invited colleagues from other agencies in Westchester County to share our experience. Short-term approaches demand constant discussion so that formulations remain sharp and therapy does not deteriorate into a superficial ritual.

GROUP PSYCHOTHERAPY PROGRAM

At any one time, well over 25 treatment groups of varying composition are in operation: adult and young adult groups, children's groups, parents' groups, couples' groups, and didactic groups. We do not regard this simply as a practical means of handling an expanding patient population; we recommend group therapy more often because we believe it is the best possible treatment for the patient than because it is the only one available. Every member of our professional staff possesses or is in the process of acquiring group skills. Once a strong group therapy program has been established, it facilitates the training of new staff members who lack group therapy experience. We invite them, as well as most of our students, to become cotherapists in ongoing groups. A weekly staff workshop provides continuous case conferences which dissect the unfolding experience of representative groups at the clinic.

It has become customary for staff members to work at least one evening a week, enabling the majority of our adult groups to meet after working hours. In addition to accommodating patients who cannot take time off from work on a regular basis, evening groups have the further advantage of serving a heterogeneous male and female patient population, rather than being limited to unemployed housewives.

Since we have a relatively large number of groups, there is less concern about enforcing time limits; but each individual's needs are periodically reviewed. Group therapy provides a means of offering further treatment to individuals for whom short-term therapy does not constitute a sufficient intervention.

REHABILITATION AND DAY-HOSPITAL PROGRAMS

Several years ago we became concerned with the fact that many psychotic patients were being served in a fragmented, nonsystematic fashion that inadvertently had fostered excessive morbidity, chronicity, and invalidism. Services of a more comprehensive nature seemed needed for their more stubborn psychological and social needs; conventional treatment services were inappropriate, ineffective, or insufficient. Too many individuals with psychotic illnesses, acute and chronic, had been unable to connect with existing services, even though these were easily accessible and well publicized. Others were getting desultory, frequently ineffective drug therapy in state-hospital-operated aftercare programs. The minimal, token treatment they received had not been sufficient to reduce the rate of hospitalization, let alone foster social and vocational rehabilitation.

We acknowledged that we ourselves had also been reluctant to commit much of our scarce manpower to this ostensibly less rewarding task. In the absence of clearly formulated policy, only therapists with unusual interest and patience had gravitated toward and persisted with these most difficult and often least obviously responsive individuals. For other patients, minimal supportive therapy had made little dent in feelings of incompetence and incapacity.

We concluded that these patients desperately needed a comprehensive program which provided both acute, crisis-oriented therapy and treatment modalities for rehabilitation and extended care. We developed a proposal for a multiphasic approach which could offer a continuum of meaningful services appropriate for acute, recurring, or persisting needs.[15] Particularly important, we sought to develop an attitude of positive expectancy which might in some cases generate major life changes, and in others promote greater self-sufficiency. A demonstration grant was obtained in 1970 from the New York State Department of Mental Hygiene under the 314/D program of the National Institutes of Mental Health.

The program was developed to provide continuing care for chronically hospitalized psychotic patients and emergency treatment for acutely disturbed patients who might be spared hospitalization. Distinctive components include multiple lines of communication with public hospitals to assure continuity of care; comprehensive treatment services emphasizing family and group approaches, including home visits; crisis intervention for patients and families to avert unnecessary hospitalization; active collaboration with vocational rehabilitation and employment services; training of paraprofessionals to serve as liaison agents, expediters, counselors, and co-therapists in a multiplicity of roles needed in the social rehabilitation of patients; keeping track of once-psychotic patients within the catchment area, so that they can be periodically reassessed; and development of an active case-finding program to locate nonfunctioning psychotic individuals in the community who are as yet unidentified by community resources.

Several of these features deserve emphasis. We put much effort into the development of good working relationships with many echelons of the public and private hospitals which receive patients from our catchment area. We attempted to participate in discharge planning early in the course of hospitalization. We offered an alternative to lengthy hospitalization or transfer to more distant state institutions.

Following discharge from the hospital, a member of our staff sees the patient and his family immediately (a home visit is routine), since we believe this is the most critical period for both patient and family.

A major therapeutic emphasis is on the learning and rehearsal of social skills; group and family therapies therefore constitute an important component of the program. We emphasize flexibility in a multiphasic approach: crisis intervention and pharmacotherapy during an acute psychotic episode; day treatment; continuing group, family, or individual therapy; afternoon and evening socialization groups; and visits on a less frequent basis as patients recover.

The Day Hospital

As our rehabilitation program developed, it became clear that there were many individuals who initially required a more structured, supportive daily program. The day hospital was a natural outgrowth, but the original grant enabled us to develop only a half-day program staffed in large part by volunteers. Within 2 years, the value of this program in maintaining in the community patients who otherwise would have been rehospitalized in state hospitals became incontrovertible. It was then that the community mental health board agreed to seek further county funds for an expanded full-day program, with sufficient staff to develop a therapeutic community approach and a variety of treatment and activity groups.

The lack of hospital beds within our district has been a conspicuous deficiency of our total program. Until the local hospital introduces a psychiatric inpatient service, we must depend upon publicly supported beds outside our catchment area. As the day program has developed, the need for psychiatric beds becomes less pressing. Surprisingly few patients require rehospitalization, and when this becomes unavoidable, the duration of hospitalization is usually measured in weeks rather than months or years, since both patients and hospital staff know that our day program is waiting for the patient to return. Increasing numbers of acutely psychotic patients are managed in the day program without being hospitalized at all.

Over 95 percent of the patients in the rehabilitation and day programs are psychotic and more than 75 percent are schizophrenic. Analysis of our evaluative data indicates that over 70 percent of the patients can be helped to function in the community. Most of the treatment failures can be described as follows: patients with alcoholism or addiction as additional problems; unstable drifters, unanchored in the community, who disappear within the first weeks after entering the program; patients who are markedly unrelated, disorganized, or unmotivatable if family or friends cannot provide support and shelter. These findings have suggested the need for additional programs such as a halfway house and an alcoholism program.

SERVICES FOR CHILDREN

The children's program was redesigned several years ago so that we might provide prompter and more effective services. This entailed changes both in the timing and the thrust of our response.

Counseling Services

In developing rapid evaluative and short-term techniques for children, greater difficulties are initially encountered than in introducing a similar program for adults.[14] Particularly before a clinic has conceptualized problem categories that encompass its patient population, children's problems are less easily triaged on the basis of a short initial contact. The child himself, often referred by disgruntled educators or enforcement officers, may be reticent, but this need not discourage a direct approach. Information from parents, school, and other informants can be collated without resorting to the inefficiencies of the "holy trinity" approach (evaluation and conferencing by psychiatrist, psychologist, and social worker) that consumes as much time as would a brief therapeutic intervention.

As our system presently functions, the applicant's needs are immediately explored in a probing telephone contact by a senior member of our staff. New applications are critically examined at a weekly children's coordinating conference, where efforts are immediately under way to categorize the nature of the problem and conceptualize the range of possible interventions. Cases are assigned for what is judged to be the most appropriate therapeutic modality and are reviewed 4–6 weeks later.

Paralleling our approach to adults, our aim is to handle about one third of the patients accepted for treatment in each of the following ways:

1. Crisis intervention or short-term therapy for children with apparently delimited problems, or those unamenable to more extensive therapy.
2. Therapeutic groups for children of all ages. We have been developing more specialized small group approaches for groups of three to four children and their parents. These groups utilize role playing, dramatics, gestalt approaches, and more traditional talk therapies. The parents and the children are seen in separate groups and periodically the groups meet together.
3. Longer-term therapies for children with multiple dimensions of disturbance or multiple levels of deficit. These children often come from fragmented or multiproblem families.

Sometimes the most fitting therapeutic approach can be established only by a trial of short-term therapy. As with adults, we attempt to reserve more extensive procedures for the more disturbed patients.[7,8]

We would like to be able to reach more children at the time of crisis, before their problems have been compounded. Early identification of a child's problem increases the likelihood that short-term, preventively oriented approaches will have sufficient impact. We will not permit children to languish on a waiting list.

Since limited staff precludes the possibility of long-term individual therapy for all the children who need it, we are at the same time supplementing our resources by training volunteers for long-term "relationship" therapy. Having observed with great interest the successes of others in training college students as companion counselors for adolescents,[16] we are also exploring these possibilities with some of our local colleges.

The other crucial aspect of our therapeutic redesign is the redefinition of who is the patient. The attitudes and actions of adults are frequently instrumental in setting the stage for a child's problems and, perhaps unwittingly, perpetuating them. Parents, relatives, and teachers can respond more readily to appeals to reason, and they are better positioned to interrupt vicious cycles (or conversely, to undermine any gains the child achieves in therapy). We are convinced that work with the family system often is more expedient and more productive than directly treating the child. Whenever possible we conceptualize children's problems in terms of the family or social system which generates or reinforces them; we are increasingly on the lookout for opportunities to alter that system at a point of maximum impact. Treating the family can change a pathogenic system before it adversely affects other children in the family who have not yet been compromised.

A systems approach[17,18] necessitates close collaboration with key components of the child's life, particularly school personnel, community agencies, and town officials. We have been developing consultative relationships with school personnel, including principals and teachers as well as psychologists and social workers. Our aims are both to achieve a better exchange of information and to enhance skills of those who are the de facto providers of mental health services for the great majority of troubled children who cannot, and in many cases should not, be treated in mental health clinics.[9,19]

Other forms of collaboration deal more explicitly with early detection of learning and behavior problems in elementary school and preschool children. A psychologist on our staff has served as consultant to a day-care program, working with the mothers of children who are beginning to manifest behavioral disturbances. He provides consultation to their principals and teachers. In the elementary and high schools, he meets regularly with guidance counselors, psychologists, and social workers, focusing upon individual cases and work with groups. Several school psychologists have been helped to develop time-limited counseling groups of their own for parents of underachieving first and second graders; a study revealed that these children made significant learning gains as compared with a group of controls. We have also been helping psychologists and social workers to develop counseling groups for children who have academic and behavior problems. We have helped launch a project in which high-school students will tutor first and second graders. The objective of each of these endeavors is to introduce models which can be adopted and maintained by school staff.

Therapeutic Nursery School

The therapeutic nursery school was developed 6 years ago, when a computerized analysis of requests for therapy in the preceding year revealed that 38 out of 620 applications were for children between the ages of 3 and 5. An exploration of community resources for this age group indicated an almost total void, both public and private, in all of Westchester County. Professionals throughout the county followed with interest our efforts to develop a daily therapeutic milieu. The aim was to provide maximal psychological and social services for children as young as 3 years and to help those with serious emotional handicaps to reach a successful school adjustment leading to a transition to a normal school setting.

The program presently serves 12 to 14 children between 3 to 5 years of age, referred from such sources as prekindergarten programs and day-care centers. In order to qualify, these children must have severe disruptive disturbances which cannot be handled in ordinary settings. Many are regressive, destructive, and hyperactive. Others are withdrawn and immobile. The children attend the therapeutically oriented educational program daily, generally for at least 1 year. Concurrently, parents have regular individual or group therapy sessions and are invited to participate in the nursery to learn how to find better ways of handling their children's difficulties. Many of the children come from multiproblem families which need much assistance. After graduating, the majority of the children have been able to enter normal school settings, where they are periodically followed by the nursery staff.

The therapeutic nursery also serves as an ideal resource for providing diagnostic evaluations based on extensive observations of the child's functioning in a schoolroom setting. Additionally, it offers opportunities to develop consultative relationships with community agencies, such as child-care and prekindergarten programs, as well as teachers in kindergarten and first grade. The nursery has been an important training resource in the community. A formal proposal was developed several years ago for its expansion to serve 24 children. Extending the age range to incorporate early elementary grades has also been contemplated. Although there is widespread community agreement about the urgent need for expanded services, a suitable funding mechanism remains to be found.

SATELLITE PROGRAMS

In reaching out to the community, we have found that it is advantageous to develop satellite programs located in areas which otherwise do not sufficiently make use of available mental health resources. Six years ago a computerized study of the demographical and geographical characteristics of our population pinpointed several subgroups that were not receiving services commensurate with their needs.

The majority of the 9.5 percent of families in New Rochelle with incomes under $3000 are black. Most of these families are clustered in ghetto areas containing large housing projects, some of which are within sight of areas of affluence. We singled out the census tract with the lowest per capita income in New Rochelle. Poor black families in this area were not sufficiently using our services, and those families who did tended to drop out from therapy most quickly. Discussions with black community leaders elicited the information that many of the people in their neighborhood felt alienated from what they assumed was a white, middle-class clinic, even though considerable effort had been made to change this inaccurate image. This community wanted a neighborhood clinic it could more readily identify as its own, one which would be staffed by black professionals.

In response to these sentiments, we started a pilot project in 1967, initially with limited funds, in the basement of a housing project. The staff was headed by a black psychiatrist and a black psychologist, both highly respected residents of the community. Obtaining widespread community support took time, but an even greater problem was developing a financial base that would provide adequate space, staff, and other essentials. Initial generous gifts from benefactors were not forthcoming on a recurring basis; there was a period of several years during which financing was shaky and staff and quarters insufficient. During this time, this branch clinic developed its own, largely black board of directors and continued to mobilize community support. Programs were developed that met special community needs: group therapy for children with school problems, school consultation, groups for mothers on welfare, evening and weekend services, consultation to community workers, training of indigenous paraprofessionals, and even an ambitious therapeutic summer day-camp program for disturbed youngsters. These programs were responsive to community wants, determined by a door-to-door survey in the housing project.

Two years ago, Westchester County agreed to provide additional financial support, enabling the clinic to enlarge its services. In the fall of 1971, it moved into a newly constructed neighborhood center which also houses a day-care program for preschool children, a community action program, a branch of the youth bureau, legal aid services, and public health services. The clinic now is ideally situated to provide consultative services to these agencies.

The Larchmont-Mamaroneck branch was also developed on an initially modest basis, with part-time staff. Studies had shown that individuals from this community, particularly children, were so deterred by inadequate suburban public transportation that most had failed to keep more than a few appointments at the hard-to-reach New Rochelle office. Since initial staffing was modest, services at first were limited to school-age children, a group this community regarded as its greatest concern. Emphasis was placed upon developing collaborative relationships with school staff, an approach facilitated by the unusual receptiveness of the Larchmont-Mamaroneck school system. Counseling groups were developed in the elementary and high schools, conducted by clinic staff; guidance personnel, and in some cases teachers, served as cotherapists. In addition to the direct help provided for the children, we were able to train many members of the school staff, who now conduct their own groups.

From the start, this clinic experimented with training and utilizing paraprofessional therapists with a variety of backgrounds. Welfare workers, for example, work voluntarily in the clinic at night, seeing patients under supervision and acquiring counseling skills which they can later apply in working with their own clients.

As the clinic staff, paid and volunteer, has expanded, services have been extended to patients of all ages. A major emphasis continues to be the provision of consultation services. Two years ago this clinic was instrumental in highlighting the need for a program for youthful drug abusers in this community. Several staff members helped to develop a proposal for a special outreach program which was funded by the New York State Narcotics Addiction Control Commission. After helping to recruit a staff, the clinic then provided consultation and training for it.

DRUG-ABUSE PROGRAMS

When we began dealing with the addiction problem on a large scale 5 years ago, we soon realized that conventional therapeutic resources had severe limitations, particularly as drug use became more malignant. We developed a collaborative relationship with an ex-addict program in our district, engendering mutual consultation and referral of patients. We also initiated an outpatient methadone detoxification program, but insufficient treatment resources in our community for the growing number of heroin addicts whom we detoxified (one or two per week) resulted in an enormous relapse rate. At the same time, we began a series of meetings with community leaders, who were by then so alarmed by the drug problem that their active cooperation was not difficult to enlist. In a black neighborhood, a door-to-door survey we conducted revealed that most residents regarded addiction as their number one problem.

We explored several possible treatment programs that we might develop, including methadone maintenance. When large-scale funding suddenly became available for the latter, many of us had already begun to believe that methadone would be the only effective treatment for hard-core heroin addicts. The community response was more mixed.

The issue of obtaining community consensus in such matters is certainly more complicated than some have claimed.[9,20] Experienced clinicians were in conflict about which therapeutic approach was most promising. Community leaders were even more divided, but many were so desperate that they were ready to try anything. We conducted community meetings, informing people about the rationale for methadone, its advantages and drawbacks. Some black community leaders were resistive, and we had to allay their fears that methadone could cause brain damage.

Far thornier were the charges that methadone would become a means of pacifying otherwise "objectionable" minority elements in the community. Community sentiment as a whole supported our proposal for a methadone program.

Our first satellite methadone clinic, started in a storefront in central New Rochelle in 1970, admitted 125 heroin addicts for outpatient detoxification and methadone maintenance in a period of less than 3 months. The magnitude of the heroin problem in the suburbs had exceeded everyone's wildest fears. A second satellite program was introduced the following year, and its enrollment reached capacity almost as quickly.

Strikingly parallel to the experiences first reported by Dole, Nyswander, and Warner[21] in New York City, our methadone clinics have achieved a success rate of over 80 percent. This is established by "hard" criteria such as clean urine samples, no further arrests, and resuming functioning at work, home, and/or school. Major program emphases are helping addicts to attain probationary status with the courts, to straighten out other legal difficulties, and to secure jobs. Other addicts require more extensive psychotherapeutic interventions. Family and group therapies are provided when necessary by the professional and paraprofessional staffs. These staffs have become well acquainted with key members of the community, particularly judges, police officers, and employers. Still unsolved is the problem of the recidivist patient, who continues addiction to alcohol, pills, or other harmful substances. We are attempting to develop additional therapeutic modalities to reach these patients.

EMERGING PROBLEMS AND PROSPECTS OF THE COMMUNITY MENTAL HEALTH CLINIC

In the remainder of this chapter, I shall discuss some more general issues which face community mental health clinics. As we enter a period of rapid and fundamental change, opportunities to develop more comprehensive, multifaceted, community-related services have generated excitement and challenge. Concurrently, effective coordination, planning, and evaluation cannot be neglected.

While some clinics are experiencing unprecedented growth, others are already operating more defensively, in some instances less concerned with innovation and experimentation than with mere survival. During this period of economic crisis, merely preserving intact what already exists poses no small problem for many clinics. To sustain vitality and effectiveness, however, even those clinics which are forced to retrench must maintain a process of self-examination and identity redefinition. They must eliminate outworn institutional practices legitimized primarily by tradition, and struggle to reshape programs in order that they may best answer community needs.

Whether in a stage of expansion or just holding their own, clinics must seek continuing professional growth and high standards of excellence and creative aspiration. Staff must be challenged to embrace new, more appropriate professional roles which better reflect community mental health objectives. This implies an ongoing discussion of the staff's perception of its own professional needs and wants. We must remind ourselves that professionals sometimes gravitate toward practices and organizational structures that serve their own needs better than those of the community. These issues must become open and negotiable. The clinic should be an evolving organism that is open to change.

Stimulating clinic staff to function at a high level of purpose and esprit is made more difficult when worsening fiscal pressures, seemingly indifferent to our concerns about providing quality service, periodically threaten to decimate vitally needed programs. The procrustean bed into which budgetary squeezes would force us must not be allowed to shrivel our growing edge. Otherwise our programs can quickly deteriorate into a new institutionalism which stultifies the needs of patients, staff, and community.

I can only touch upon some of these issues in the most cursory fashion. I shall focus particularly upon (1) staff development and role expansion, (2) the community stake, (3) financial shortages and the government partner, and (4) future planning for comprehensive public health services.

Staffing Realities

Sometimes it takes harsh exigencies to foster experimentation that could as well have been stimulated by less practical concerns. It has not been too many years since social workers, psychologists, and other mental health professionals were relegated to subsidiary positions in the mental health hierarchy. Regardless of their capabilities and talents, it was the psychiatrist who reigned supreme. Particularly in medical settings, the psychiatrist had been granted the role of psychotherapist, with all the prestige, authority, and therapeutic magic that role commands. Other professionals were expected to serve in what often amounted to adjunctive roles. Social workers, for example, did intake interviews, social histories, counseling of families of hospitalized patients, or environmental manipulation. In settings where this role limitation has been unfeasible, the psychiatrist was expected at the very least to conceptualize, supervise, and assume responsibility for treatment.

Was this role separation necessitated by clinical considerations, or did it reflect more archaic concerns? Many mental health professionals already possess, and most others can acquire, a level of diagnostic acumen and psychotherapeutic sophistication which permits them to function with more authority, independence, and charisma. A professional caste system, finally changing in some settings, may simply reflect the inertia of institutions (or an antifeminist bias), not inherent limitations in nonmedical therapists.

The objectives of psychotherapy are being redefined within a broader social context. Mental health clinics must capitalize upon the therapeutic capabilities of every member of the staff in order to achieve their expanded mission. The era of the traditional, slow-paced mental health clinic, oriented toward the middle-class patient and therefore not overburdened by large numbers of applicants, is becoming a relic of the past.

Those who refer patients to mental health clinics must be made aware of this changing philosophy. Many patients are still referred by professionals with the gratuitous request that "the patient must be seen by a psychiatrist." We must make it understood that psychotherapy in public health settings takes many forms, only one of which is the uncovering, reconstructive therapy for which psychiatrists may have been more specifically trained. Serving the more functionally compromised members of the community, in a variety of ways, has become a higher priority for mental health clinics than serving the self-dissatisfied but functionally intact.[9,22-24] This calls for techniques of social rehabilitation, group process, environmental restructuring, and systems change, often in preference to strategies of traditional psychotherapy. And the latter, in community settings, have become more oriented toward strengthening the healthy portions of the ego and focusing upon the patient's adaptive skills. Rather than peeling off multiple layers of resistance and uncovering unresolved childhood conflicts or their instictual precursors, psychotherapy in clinic settings focuses upon maladaptive behavior patterns and problem-solving techniques. Mental health professionals in every discipline have had, or should obtain, training in adaptational psychotherapy.[25] The psychiatrist can be called upon as a consultant, when there is a need for his special skills, such as differential diagnosis, medical or neurological evaluation, and pharmacotherapy. For that matter, his knowledge of complex psychodynamic patterns is increasingly shared by well-trained professionals in other disciplines.

Our clinic is introducing therapists in every discipline to procedures once regarded as the exclusive domain of the psychiatrist, a species increasingly hard to capture and support. The lure of private practice, and competition with academic institutions, makes it difficult to retain all but the most dedicated psychiatrists in positions other than those of leadership. We find that most applicants for vacant psychiatric positions are newly trained graduates, hardly the equal of many of our more experienced nonmedical staff. We are training all staff members to do mental status examinations and to make initial diagnoses, which can be confirmed by a psychiatrist when necessary. Nor are psychiatrists always needed for emergency examinations, evaluation of suicidal risk, or assessment of the need for hospitalization.

For the last few years, I have conducted for all new staff members an annual workshop which deals with psychotropic drugs. We examine therapeutic indications, mechanisms of action, side effects, and other issues. I believe that nonmedical therapists should participate in the process of considering psychotropic medication, though the ultimate decision and responsibility must be assumed by a physician.

Training of this kind enables staff members, including paraprofessionals, to make emergency home visits to acutely disturbed patients. Their mental status examinations can establish diagnoses such as acute schizophrenic episode or organic brain syndrome; they learn to outline an appropriate plan of treatment which they discuss with a psychiatrist.

Training and Use of Paraprofessional Case Aides

Increasing shortages of professionals and funds have stimulated mental health clinics to find new roles for paraprofessionals and volunteers. The guidance center first began using volunteers in paraclinical roles such as remedial reading, parent education, aides in the therapeutic nursery, and counselors in the therapeutic day camp. This last program, started 5 years ago, provided up to 40 youngsters with a summer arts and recreational program that included swimming in the backyard pools of board members.

Several years ago, we began to wonder whether we could use qualified volunteers in more ambitious capacities. We had long felt that many deprived, lonely, awkward, or socially insecure children really needed a continuing therapeutically oriented relationship with a stable adult figure, rather than traditional kinds of interpretive psychotherapy. Carefully chosen volunteers, selected from a large group of applicants, were supervised in "relationship therapy" with disturbed children or adolescents. The results were impressive and encouraged expansion of the program.

When we designed a demonstration program for the rehabilitation of psychotic patients, an important component was the training of paraprofessionals. Not only would they be trained to work as individual and group therapists, but they would help patients to become reoriented in the community and to utilize essential services such as vocational rehabilitation programs. Novice psychotherapists (such as first-year psychiatric residents) sometimes achieve a remarkable level of success with disturbed patients because of their unfettered imagination, enthusiasm, optimism, and unwillingness to be discouraged by poor prognostic indicators. Working within a structured, supervised setting, paraprofessionals can achieve impressive results with some of the most difficult patients. Gradually they develop impressive professional-level skills.

Continuing Education and Staff Esprit

Situated in an attractively located suburb in a major metropolitan area, we have no difficulty recruiting highly qualified professionals, many of whom already have impressive abilities. I doubt whether clinics in most parts of the country have comparable pools of talent from which to choose. Changing perspectives and goals, however, demand a continuing process of acquiring and modifying therapeutic skills. Equally important, staff esprit is nourished by varying forms of stimulation, including the challenge of new ideas and undertakings. Important to the success of a clinic's program is the development of a self-image as an organization with creative strivings and an expanding technology. Seeking intellectual and social challenges generates a sense of aspiration and commitment among staff. We try to avoid the incrustations of mechanical routine.

Academic settings seem to possess a special mystique. Psychiatrists in particular will accept positions offering lower salaries and fewer creative opportunities in preference to jobs in community clinics where there can be better possibilities to grow professionally. Academic settings have no monopoly on excellence or discovery. But mental health clinics have to work harder to project an image which attracts top-level staff. This is one telling argument for larger, more comprehensive clinics which can offer a variety of professional interaction and stimulation.

We offer many workshops: group therapy, family therapy, pharmacotherapy, brief therapy. Each of our special programs has ongoing staff conferences in which much teaching occurs. "T"-groups provide another kind of training experience. Individual supervision is provided to all junior staff, and to others when needed. Our many training programs offer staff members the special stimulation of teaching. Probably most important, though less tangible, is the day-to-day contact and cross fertilization among energetic, creative, committed staff members who value the freedom to work independently, explore new ideas, and share them with an interested professional community. The importance of developing an environment that promotes professional growth cannot be overstressed. The stringency of government funding sources in disallowing expenditures for in-service training is ultimately much costlier if staff potential is insufficiently realized.

Polyphonic Voices

A changing clinic must redefine organization and objectives. The Community Mental Health Act has provided a general sense of direction: centers serving defined catchment areas, providing essential services, seeking a broad community base, and responsive to the community's most pressing mental health needs. The ingredients vary considerably in different settings, reflecting diverse concerns: What does the community want, and how can this be ascertained? How is the broad national mandate translated into specific guidelines by the state department of mental hygiene and the community mental health board? With what fiscal carrot or clout? How does this mesh with the ideas of the clinic leadership, board, and staff? Differences must be mediated without consuming inordinate amounts of time and energy, as has been known to happen in some settings.

As part of the federal mandate, the consumer voice has been given particular emphasis.[20] However, obtaining a fair sampling of consumer opinion is no easy task. The most vocal community spokesmen can articulate extreme, polarized positions reflecting the viewpoint of no more than a small part of their constituencies. Their hortatory, politically tuned statements can produce devisiveness or defensiveness in community meetings. It is difficult to sift out the legitimacy of the needs of the socially disadvantaged from the impracticality or impetuosity of their spokesmen's demands for immediate action, for which neither funds nor organizational groundwork have been provided.

On the other hand, it is no easy matter to mobilize continuing interest from all low-income groups which are part of the clinic's constituency. Some of their representatives do not have clearly articulated viewpoints; others are not sufficiently involved to attend meetings regularly. In our efforts to develop a community council, the unevenness of representation from the community we serve has been disheartening. Yet the council lacks the funds to employ a community organizer who could ferret out more community representation while informing the different subgroups in the community about important issues. The very government agencies which mandate community participation have failed, in this instance, to anticipate sources of funds which would make it a viable concept. In consequence, the mental health coordinating council which we helped to organize in our catchment area is weighted too heavily with representatives from local health, education, and welfare agencies. The community mental health board is delegating increasing responsibility to the council; it must approve proposals for new programs before they can be considered for government funds, and it evaluates and coordinates existing services.

In formulating policy and suggesting new programs, the clinic director is responsible to the board of directors. Boards have also been developed for each of our satellite programs, and their composition reflects a variety of viewpoints. Proposals for new programs must be approved by our board, but public meetings open to all members of the community provide a forum for further discussions and suggestions.

Fortunately, both the New York State Department of Mental Hygiene and the Westchester Community Mental Health Board have been enunciating program objectives which we ourselves heartily embrace, e.g., defining priority target populations such as the severely disturbed, socially disadvantaged, alcoholic, and aged patients. With regard to broad policy matters, the only major point of contention has been the omission of children's services from the list of priorities, and the resulting insufficiency of funds available for the support and development of children's programs. With regard to implementation, the major issues revolve around financing: the proportion of government support, to be discussed more fully below, and the lack of flexibility permitted in changing job lines, allocating expenditures for staff training, and the like. Although the funds are provided by New York State, it is the community mental health board to whom responsibility is delegated for regulation of clinic activities on the local level. It is here that our organizational structure as a private agency with its own board of directors is particularly beneficial. A private clinic can develop independent viewpoints which its board can negotiate with government policy makers. The position of government-operated institutions is considerably weaker.

The Fiscal Maelstrom

Funding under the Community Mental Health Centers Act is initially generous; surpluses have been exploited by some large institutions as a means of supporting other services and plugging financial gaps.[22,26] Paradoxically, our program embraces most of the goals specified by the federal legislation, but we are unlikely ever to have a share of the funds it provides to develop new community programs.

Several years ago, when we contemplated submission of a proposal, we encountered some major obstacles. First, *relatively* speaking, Westchester County has a multiplicity of (unfortunately fragmented) mental health services which in total exceeds the resources of many other areas of New York State, particularly New York City. It appeared that the regional office of the National Institutes of Health would assign Westchester proposals a low priority. The most evident need, *relative* to the rest of the state, was for a better coordinated network of services. The community mental health board concentrated upon promoting coordinating structures in the six catchment areas. These may eventually assume the formal status of community mental health centers, but probably without the help of federal funds. In our district, another major obstacle was our local hospital's temporizing about developing an inpatient service which would supply that essential center component which we are not well situated or disposed to develop. The hospital agrees in principle that an inpatient unit is needed, but the new building which will house it will not be constructed for another 4 or 5 years.

There were even more troubling concerns which made us look upon the funding concept of the Community Mental Health Centers Act with scepticism. This legislation assumes that, once needed new programs are launched with the assistance of federal seed money, alternative funding sources at the local and state level will quickly become available to sustain these programs. The federal share diminishes rapidly: After 2 years it is 60 percent; from the fifth through the eighth years it is 30 percent. Many clinics have been unable to develop sufficient local support to take the place of diminishing federal funds,[22,24,26] and in some cases their very survival is in jeopardy.

Local clinics thus find themselves caught in the middle as federal, state, county, and local governments continue the evasive game of determining who will pick up the tab. Local government budgets are reaching their ceilings and local legislators are loath or unable to impose additional taxes. Urgent pleas for the support of even the most vital services receive a sympathetic hearing, but local administrators insist there is little that they can do: The responsibility for funding is really at a different level of government, not theirs. The Revenue Sharing Act may make this buck-passing even worse.

The politics of government funding generally is not concerned with long-range realities. This inveterate shortsightedness leaves clinics scrambling madly for new funding sources every few years. In the process it generates some meritorious programs with a brief life span. The cost of implementing comprehensive mental health programs continues to escalate; ultimately the federal government will have to accept its responsibility to provide continuing support, either directly or by some form of national insurance. Otherwise the temptation for each level of government to defer responsibility to another will be almost irresistible. Broad policy guidelines should be evolved by the National Institutes of Mental Health and by the professional societies.

When costs began escalating at their steepest rates several years ago, it became apparent that the Guidance Center would have to find new sources of funds. Hitherto the funds for the clinic had been raised primarily by an active, dedicated board of directors and a large general membership. The latter presently numbers over 400. Although these individuals continue to mount a vigorous, diversified fund-raising campaign, one of the most successful in Westchester County, the monies raised simply can no longer keep pace with the inflationary spiral; they cannot maintain existing services, let alone finance new programs. The board's contribution has represented a sharply decreasing proportion of our total budget.

Inevitably, the major source of funds for new or expanded programs has been government grants which do not require the clinic to raise any portion of the costs. The New York State Narcotics Addiction Control Commission meets all costs in the methadone programs which are not covered by medicaid fees, themselves substantial. Our programs for rehabilitating chronically ill patients were originally financed by a special grant. In our experience these programs for more chronically disturbed patients eventually generate sufficient medicaid fees to cover a considerable part of their cost. Government funding must provide the remainder.

I have come to realize that one often has little choice in the timing of one's programmatic goals. The following narrative provides an illustration.

For the last two years we have been vainly struggling to expand day treatment services for children, always a major concern of our board and our community. The therapeutic nursery has developed a model for day treatment services which has generated much enthusiasm in the community. Its staff, increasingly expert, has been able to provide sophisticated training for growing numbers of professionals and paraprofessionals throughout the county. Expanding this program, and eventually providing services for children up to fourth grade, had seemed the logical next step for which there has been broad community support. Yet when a proposal was developed and submitted to several potential funding sources a few years ago, no money could be found.

At around the same time, federal funds suddenly became available in abundance from a new division of the National Institutes of Mental Health for the development of alcoholism programs. In 1973, over $100 million* will be available for this purpose. In the past, the thought of developing an alcoholism program, although this is another high priority in our district, has generated far less enthusiasm among our staff and our board.

When funds suddenly became available, our local mental health coordinating council appointed a subcommittee to examine the magnitude of the alcohol problem and to come up with some recommendations. Statistics were obtained from the department of welfare, local courts, police, clergymen, physicians, and public health nurses. To no one's surprise, they convincingly documented the fact that there were several thousand unrehabilitated alcoholics in the district. Some 10 percent of the applicants to the Guidance Center had alcohol problems; in the absence of

---

*Six times as much as has been specifically allocated for children's programs.[27]

special services for this population, therapeutic results were poorer than for any other defined category of patients served.

The mental health coordinating council urged the local hospital to sponsor an alcoholism program and offered every possible form of assistance. The hospital expressed interest but declined to accept responsibility for developing the proposal. When it became evident that the Guidance Center was the only other agency in our district which possessed this capability, we found ourselves faced with a troubling decision. This was not a program which had previously fired our imagination; yet the need was unmistakable. After a series of soul-searching discussions with our staff and board, we agreed to assume the responsibility and we submitted a proposal for an ambitious satellite program, incorporating crisis teams, partial hospitalization, and public education.

Given the choice, the so-called consumers in our community as well as our own board would have overwhelmingly opted for expanding the children's program. Turnouts at public meetings, such as those chaired by the coordinating council, had been large and enthusiastic when the agenda was devoted to children's services. The mothers of schoolchildren who are in ''special'' classes are particularly organized and vocal. In contrast, attendance at meetings devoted to the alcoholism problem was disappointing. Does this signify a smaller constituency, or is it a reflection of the lack of organization of alcoholics and their families *in this community,* or their unwillingness to so identify themselves? Regardless of articulated community wants, it is the availability of federal money which has in this instance been decisive—the need for an alcoholism program itself being clear. In the meantime, the quest for funding for a day treatment program for children continues.

Thus, realistic clinic directors, working in conjunction with board, staff, and community, must proceed on two levels: persisting in the search for funds to support programs the community especially desires, while at the same time integrating the reality of present fiscal patterns with the development of programs for which there is legitimate need. We must define a spectrum of community mental health needs. We may weight these needs in terms of what the system would prefer, but it is probably a mistake to become too insistent upon the *order* in which objectives must be realized. We all have our subjective professional preferences, but there are challenges and satisfactions in developing creative programs for a variety of priority patient populations, whether they be the aged, the schizophrenic, the alcoholic, or the maladjusted schoolchild. One must, with community support, capitalize upon opportunities as they emerge, after making certain that programs can be sustained when initial funding is exhausted.

Living with present political realities does not mean that we passively accept them. A pragmatic approach does not prevent us from redoubling our efforts to bring persuasive pressure upon the federal government to change funding policies.

Since the cost of maintaining psychotic patients in the community is a fraction of the cost of hospitalization in state institutions, government agencies are more likely to provide total continuing support for these programs. Indeed, were mental health clinics really to serve those populations for whom they had originally been established,[22,24] the expenditures for state institutions, particularly in a state like New York, would be so reduced that the government could reallocate these funds for supporting local programs. This has been the experience in California, and it is a long-range objective which must be pursued in other states.

Private insurance mechanisms could be another major source of clinic funds. At present most insurance plans are heavily biased in the direction of inpatient services; many reimburse only for the services of a physician. These senseless insurance limitations are responsible for the excessive use of hospitalization in many institutions which depend upon inpatient fees to cover the deficits of outpatient services. For these institutions, shifting the emphasis to outpatient services such as day treatment would require a comparable financial incentive. The costs of psychiatric hospitalization in most institutions in the metropolitan New York area exceed $1000 per week. Many insurance plans cover the greatest part of this cost. The cost of day treatment at the Guidance Center (which most patients are not expected to pay) is about one tenth of this. Nonetheless most insurance plans will not reimburse the Guidance Center, a free-standing clinic, for services which prevent or shorten hospitalization. In this instance, Westchester County agreed to provide a portion of the cost, recognizing that the day program is both cheaper and in many instances more effective than hospitalization in publicly supported hospital beds.

If the above discussion seems to represent a disproportionately heavy emphasis upon financing, it reflects one clinic director's preoccupation with this vexing subject, at a time when many clinics are experiencing the most severe financial crises in their history. Discussions of objectives alone are futile when these cannot be launched or, more important, sustained. It is often pragmatics which spell the difference between vision and reality.

Future Planning Amid Present Uncertainties

A few years ago, I used to take pride in appearing at our annual membership meeting spouting statistics which demonstrated that we were increasing diagnostic and therapeutic services at a rate of 5–10 percent each year. This seemed a tangible way of documenting our increasing contribution to the mental health of the community. At present, I find these continuing increments in the provision of direct services less a source of satisfaction than a cause for concern. Obviously we cannot continue expanding at this rate indefinitely. Nonetheless, community needs continue to surface, and there is little doubt that the numbers we serve are a mere fraction of those in need of help.

Allocating scarce resources requires a broad public health perspective. Where are the pockets of most serious psychic dysfunction, and how do these relate to socioeconomic dis-ease? Do the major sources of referral reflect the greatest need from a public health viewpoint? How many dysfunctional schizophrenics, alcoholics, elderly patients, and children with thwarted emotional growth are concealed from professional view, perhaps yet unidentified by the network of professional services? Where are the psychotic individuals who seldom emerge from their households, where they languish and compound the handicaps of their maladaptive life patterns? Who in the community can help us reach these people? Upon whom will our direct therapeutic intervention have the greatest impact? How can we identify and treat, or remove "emotional contaminants?"[2] If we cannot offer services to all in need, which individuals and which families need our help most, both from their point of view, and from that of the total community? Should we not give preference to individuals upon whom the welfare of others depends, e.g., parents of a disturbed child, when there is a possibility of thus helping others in the family?

These rhetorical questions suggest one professional's viewpoint. A community clinic ought first to serve those with major needs, particularly when this can make a difference for the patient and for those around him. These individuals often remain concealed in the community, and they resist help when it is offered. It is frequently the less disturbed therapy seekers who enthusiastically, indeed determinedly, request assistance. The clinic must reach out resourcefully to find and motivate the often unidentified and initially skeptical patient. Effectuating this depends upon developing a multifaceted network of human services, both to find those who need assistance and to share the mammoth task of helping them. The mental health clinic, which cannot treat everyone, must become a training and facilitating resource for professional and nonprofessional care givers in the community.

Since the relative benefits of therapy, to patients and the community, are yet to be established, the clinic must maintain an open, experimental attitude. Short-term therapy of individuals in adaptive crises may achieve preventive goals, circumventing the development of more refractory psychopathology. This is a piece of the clinic's mission. Early detection of childhood malfunction and interruption of vicious circles which reinforce feelings of inadequacy and failure are other high-priority preventive services. Early detection and effective community-based treatment of individuals with decompensating psychotic illness are high-priority tasks which many clinics have abandoned in favor of less exhausting ones. Treatment of alcoholics and addicts is another taxing but critical clinic responsibility. Treatment of chronically impaired individuals whose prospects of regaining self-sufficiency are less sanguine cannot be ignored because to do so relegates these unfortunate individuals to the unhappy status of outcasts in nontherapeutic state institutions. Developing practical, multiphasic treatment and resocialization techniques which sustain patients in the community is another major clinic responsibility.

Community mental health must redefine traditional aims and strategies of psychotherapy, placing greatest emphasis upon social functioning in the community. We must think more and more in systems terms, focusing upon as many as possible of the critical components: the socioeconomic ecology of the community, forces of convulsive social change in the hitherto tranquil suburbs, and an emerging fraternity of helping agents within once-overlooked and stereotyped institutions such as the police, welfare, and courts, as well as the community action groups seeking change from outside the system.

The next few years will probably be a period more of consolidation than expansion of services at the Guidance Center. Programs which fail to meet expectations will be critically scrutinized, redirected, and recast. We will continue to search for funds for the expansion of vital children's services, emphasizing collaboration with schools and development of day treatment programs for more dysfunctional youngsters. The development of an inpatient service in our neighboring hospital will probably take another 4 or 5 years, and when this is achieved we look forward to developing the alliance which will enable us to provide the full spectrum of community mental health services.

REFERENCES

1. US Department of Health, Education and Welfare: Staffing of free-standing outpatient psychiatric clinics. Biometry Branch Survey and Reports Section, Stastical Note 56, 1971

2. Bellak L: Community mental health as a branch of public health. In Bellak L, Barten HH (eds): Progress in Community Mental Health, vol I. New York, Grune & Stratton, 1969

3. Caplan G: An Approach to Community Mental Health. New York, Grune & Stratton, 1961

4. Caplan G: The Theory and Practice of Mental Health Consultation. New York, Basic Books, 1970

5. Ryan W: Distress in the city: Essays on the design and administratopn of urban mental health services. Cleveland, Case Western Reserve University, 1969

6. Wolkon GH: Crisis theory, the application for treatment, and dependency. Compr Psychiatry 13:459–464, 1972

7. Eisenberg L: Child psychiatry: The past quarter century. Am J Orthopsychiatry 39:389–401, 1969

8. Levitt EE: Research on psychotherapy with children. In Bergin A E, Garfield S L (eds): Handbook of Psychotherapy and Behavior Change. New York, Wiley, 1971

9. Zusman J: Community psychiatry in 1970: Some successes and failures. Psychiatr. Q 44:687–705, 1970

10. Jacobson G: The briefest psychiatric encounter: Acute effects of evaluation. Arch Gen Psychiatry 18:718–724, 1968

11. Barten HH: The 15-minute hour: Brief therapy in a military setting. Am J Psychiatry 122:565–567, 1965

12. Barten HH: The coming of age of the brief psychotherapies. In Bellak L, Barten H H (eds): Progress in Community Mental Health, vol I. New York, Grune & Stratton, 1969

13. Barten HH: Brief Therapies. New York, Behavioral Publications, 1971

14. Barten HH, Barten S: Children and Their Parents in Brief Therapy. New York, Behavioral Publications, 1973

15. Barten HH: Developing a multiphasic rehabilitation program for psychotic patients in a community mental health clinic. Psychiatr Q 47:159–174, 1973

16. Hilgard JR, Moore US: Affiliative therapy with young adolescents. J Am Acad Child Psychiatry 8:577–605, 1969

17. Bolman WM: Systems theory, psychiatry, and school phobia. Am J Psychiatry 127:25–32, 1970

18. Kelleher D: A model for integrating special educational and community mental health services. J Special Educ 2:263–272, 1968

19. Stickney SB: Schools are our community mental health centers. Am J Psychiatry 124:1407–1414, 1968

20. Bolman WM: Community control of the community mental health center. Am J Psychiatry 129:173–180, 1972

21. Dole V P, Nyswander ME, Warner A: Successful treatment of 750 criminal addicts. JAMA 206:2708–2711, 1968

22. Chu FD, Trotter S: The Mental Health Complex. Part I. Community Mental Health Centers (Nader Report). Washing-

ton DC, Center for Study of Responsive Law, 1972

23. Mora G: The relevance of history for the community mental health approach to children. Am J Psychiatry 129:408–414, 1972

24. Schwartz DA: Community mental health in 1972: An assessment. In Barten HH, Bellak L (eds): Progress in Community Mental Health, vol II. New York, Grune & Stratton, 1972

25. Draper E, Daniels R, Rada R: Adaptive psychotherapy. Compr Psychiatry 9:372–382, 1968

26. Hall CP Jr.: The economics of mental health. Hosp Community Psychiatry 21:105–110, 1970

27. Psychiatric News 7:28, 1972

Serge Lebovici, M.D.
Philippe Paumelle, M.D.

4

An Experiment in District Psychiatry in Paris:
Psychiatry for the Community and in the Community

In Europe, most psychiatry is community psychiatry: in many countries, health care is paid for by all, so that most psychiatric facilities are accessible to a public which tends to use existing services and to demand quality care.

European mental health systems, planned and financed by taxes and/or insurance plans, seem primarily geared toward the treatment of severe chronic mental dysfunction. In the United States, treatment of the mildly neurotic received more attention for a long time than management of the seriously emotionally disturbed. For the latter patients, the United States relied mostly on the mental hospital. Community mental health centers were created to bridge the gap between the mental hospital and the outpatient service. In contrast, the Europeans have generally directed their reforms toward extending the functions of the mental hospital into the community. There, community psychiatry is not considered a specialty, and the focus of effort is on organization that will assure better delivery of care.

The factors that have effected changes in the European health systems, as well as in those of the United States, emerged during World War II. They were economic changes, the need to modernize outdated hospitals, and democratization caused by wartime pressures. In the early 1950s, with the introduction of psychotropic drugs, patients were discharged into the community, where they required af-

This chapter was translated twice under the supervision of the authors and once under the auspices of the editor, with the editorial assistance of Rhoda Katzenstein. It has nevertheless retained a distinct Gallic flavor, and we finally decided to submit rather than do excessive violence to the substance. The chapter presents the innovative work of the Association of Mental Health of the 13th arrondissement in Paris. Although many of us in the United States have had experiences comparable to those of the pioneers of the 13th arrondissement, their efforts are distinct and, in some areas, unique.—L.B.

tercare. This fostered the development of sectorization, which at first was intended
to minimize staff travel while following up patients.

Sectorization involves dividing a population by geographical sections and assigning responsibility for each sector to a particular mental hospital. The mental
health team (or teams) is responsible for providing all mental health services for
the population of the area. The outstanding feature of the sectorization program
is that a given professional or professional team stays in contact with the patient
both in and out of the hospital. This prevents the gap in transmission of information which results from even the best case-record transmission. It also maintains
the patient-therapist relationship through home visits and a mobile staff.

In the move into the community, construction of new facilities has been
deemphasized. It is more economical to remodel already existing buildings to accommodate new services, and familiar structures are found to be more acceptable
to the community. With the restructuring of mental health treatment and the opening of community facilities to patients who are not chronically ill, two benefits
have been immediately evident:

1. Outpatient facilities, originally intended to provide only aftercare, are drawing
    people who ordinarily would not have sought treatment. These people feel
    particularly free to use the services, since most are eligible for treatment in
    the mental health facilities.
2. Community attitudes have changed toward greater acceptance of the mentally
    ill because the patient base has been broadened and the mental hospitals have
    become less isolated.

An experiment in district psychiatry in the 13th arrondissement of Paris provides a particularly interesting study of mental health care in and for the community in the European setting.

ORGANIZATION OF DISTRICT PSYCHIATRY IN FRANCE

In March 1960 the French government issued guidelines for establishing a
new framework for public psychiatric services; these services would be reorganized
within geographically defined districts and adapted to the psychiatric needs of the
given population. Not much happened, except in the 13th arrondissement, until
1972, when new government decrees provided concrete rules for the establishment
of these districts, their administration, and their financing. The present proposals
define a psychiatric district for adults to include approximately 70,000 inhabitants,
with one district for the psychiatric care of children and adolescents corresponding
to three adult service districts.

Among the reasons for the long delay in implementation has been the relative
discredit attached to psychiatric practices in public services in France. Those involved were themselves providing insufficient care in enormous hospitals without
any means of extending their activity. Psychoanalytic training was attracting the

best of the young psychiatrists at the same time that district psychiatry needed to develop psychiatrists with psychoanalytic training who could concentrate on psychoses and psychoanalytic practice in the community. (It was not until 1968 that psychiatry became independent of neurology in France; until then there was a sharp distinction between the teaching of psychiatry and the actual practice of psychiatry.)

Another difficulty has been that psychiatrists in private practice are somewhat reluctant to engage in public service, under what they feel to be the hand of the state, which can determine the care to be given the mentally ill.

These are some of the variants of psychiatry in France that are helpful in understanding the development of the Association of Mental Health of the 13th Arrondissement of Paris.

DISTRICT PSYCHIATRY IN THE 13TH ARRONDISSEMENT

One of the 20 administrative districts of Paris, the 13th arrondissement had been a poor quarter since the early 19th century. Balzac spoke of "marriages of the 13th arrondissement" in his novels as examples of couples not legally married; the district's population apparently did not respond to the demands of traditional morality. In *Les Misérables*, Victor Hugo described the area of the Salpêtrière, the hospital where many years later Freud studied hysteria under Charcot amid the "barrier" of hovels then inhabited by revolutionaries and criminals.

Until well after World War II, housing conditions were poor; the apartments were old and many were without the barest comforts. Besides some important iron centers and several large automobile, airplane motor, and sugar factories, the arrondissement contained small ateliers specializing in skilled craftsmanship. Despite the miserable living conditions, the population was remarkably stable. The artisans had a fairly intense social life and had organized a number of associations dealing with local problems, sports, and culture. Certain elements, however, had a particularly poor life economically and culturally, and in these areas delinquency flourished. Some of the problems of this part of the population persist, as will be seen later. In addition there remains in the quarter a "center of transit" for migrant families living in uncomfortable lodgings and waiting to be relocated.

About 10 years ago renovation in the arrondissement began, as many of the factories departed for the suburbs and large housing developments sprang up. The incoming population is of a higher economic and social level, with higher cultural aspirations, better prepared to use public services, and particularly sensitive to family conflicts, especially to school-related problems.

The arrondissement was attractive for the experiment in district psychiatry for a number of reasons. The character of the community with its combination of populations offered a variety of opportunities and lent itself to statistically viable studies. In addition, at the time, a consultation center for alcoholics and a private center for child guidance already existed.

Coordination of these activities required an original administrative structure, with a private organization functioning as a public one. The organizers of the experiment were a team of psychiatrists, many of them psychoanalytically oriented who wanted to work outside the hospital and apply their psychoanalytic experiences while continuing teaching and research under better conditions. The team included adult psychiatrists who had received their training in traditional psychiatric hospitals, and child psychiatrists who had worked together with them in a university department and were psychoanalysts, many of them teaching at the Institute of Psychoanalysis in Paris.

Development and Organization

In 1956 a consultation service for adults was opened, and 2 years later, a service for children and adolescents began operation, both functioning without hospital support. The two embryonic mental health centers were planned as an action program, with the institutions serving only as an occasional passing-through place for the patients. In 1963 a hospital for adults was opened with a maximum capacity of 175 beds—an extremely low ratio of 1 bed per 1000 inhabitants, which was considered a risk in terms of the common hospital situation in France (an average of 2.4, and in Paris 4.39, psychiatric beds per 1000 inhabitants). Thus the necessity arose to develop institutions outside the hospital: day hospitals, night services, services particularly for adults, and so on. Figure 4-1 depicts the organization of the Association of Mental Health of the 13th Arrondissement.

In 1961, a convention established the functioning of the two mental health centers, and a plan for the development of additional institutions, not yet fully realized, was adopted. Budgetary limitations have slowed the opening of new centers. The cost and usefulness of this experiment can be properly judged only in the light of those institutions deemed necessary in the plan.

Administration and Financing

The association is a private body, although subsidized and controlled by government agencies. It is administered by a council of elected and ex-officio members. Elected members include representatives of the population—mental health and social action specialists (not paid by the association), directors of social institutions, and psychiatrists working in the community in collaboration with the district team.

Ex-officio members include government people of different levels: three municipal advisors to the City of Paris, members of the commission responsible for medical-social problems, representatives of those administrations subsidizing the association, and representatives of the social agencies which play a role in mental health.

The directors, who are psychiatrists, and the administrative director report to the council and propose new initiatives (but have no authority regarding salaries,

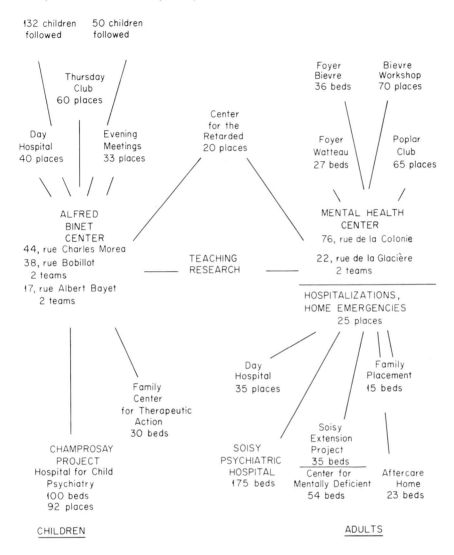

132 children   50 children
followed   followed

Thursday
Club
60 places

Foyer   Bievre
Bievre   Workshop
36 beds   70 places

Day   Evening   Center
Hospital   Meetings   for the   Foyer   Poplar
40 places   33 places   Retarded   Watteau   Club
                                20 places   27 beds   65 places

ALFRED   MENTAL HEALTH
BINET   CENTER
CENTER   76, rue de la Colonie
44, rue Charles Morea
38, rue Bobillot   TEACHING   22, rue de la Glacière
2 teams   ―――――― RESEARCH ――――――   2 teams
17, rue Albert Bayet
2 teams   HOSPITALIZATIONS,
                                                  HOME EMERGENCIES
                                                  25 places

                                Day   Family
                                Hospital   Placement
                Family   35 places   15 beds
                Center
                for Therapeutic
                Action   Soisy
                30 beds   Extension
CHAMPROSAY   SOISY   Project
PROJECT   PSYCHIATRIC   35 beds
Hospital for Child   HOSPITAL   Center for   Aftercare
Psychiatry   175 beds   Mentally Deficient Home
100 beds   54 beds   23 beds
92 places

CHILDREN   ADULTS

Fig. 4-1. Organization of the Association of Mental Health of the 13th Arrondissement.

which are aligned to those of the public services). Although private foundations can and do donate funds, financial support comes from the state, the City of Paris, and the Parisien Caisse of social security.

The administrative council therefore is a body wherein all those interested—representatives of the people who use its services, professionals, and administrators—can make decisions in common. The impact of these is limited since, in the final analysis, subsidies are accorded or refused by the administrations upon which these council members depend. The advantages of this kind of organization have been recognized recently by government authorities, who recommended creation of "district psychiatric committees," regrouping the administrations and the key personnel in local populations, such as doctors, pediatricians, policemen, judges, priests, social workers, etc. It is, however, unfortunate that the directors of the association, even though it is private, are not free to decide salaries.

The budget is twofold. The mental health centers prepare a request after discussions which, unfortunately, pay less attention to needs than to an accepted percentage of increase in spending. The institutions' budgets, on the other hand, are based on a fixed cost per day, or on the subsidy allowed each patient for a day spent in the institution. These include 14 different "prices" per day for the various institutions within the 13th arrondissement!

We have pointed out to the public powers the dangers of this double financing, which disrupts the unity and continuity of care for each patient, and have suggested instead a financing system that relates to the costs of the care offered annually to each patient. Until now, unfortunately, the administrative authorities have not wanted to abandon this classic system which differentiates between institutional and outpatient care.

We used to regret that we could not charge fees based on ability to pay, in view of modifications in the composition of the district's population. The middle-class families who have been moving into the 13th arrondissement are not only sensitive to psychiatric problems, but are prepared to use to the utmost the resources of public services. We have wondered whether they are likely to displace the socially and culturally disadvantaged who more desperately need the free service. Fortunately this fear has not been confirmed by our statistics.

These few observations explain why the originators of the experiment insisted on maintaining a strong relationship between the professional and administrative services and why the association is directed as it is. Each department is supervised by a psychiatrist, with his staff, social welfare workers, and the administrative director oriented in the same direction.

Professional Principles

At the outset, the teams insisted that the term "community psychiatry" be discarded in favor of "psychiatry in the community" to emphasize certain premises:

1. That the whole field and practice of psychiatry be included in the plan, and that reform begin with the transfer of the treating persons from the closed institutions to the common collectivity.
2. That the teams refuse to assume the functions assigned to psychiatrists within the traditional classic structure.
3. That continuity of care be of prime importance in the endeavor to reduce the

frequency and intensity of the mechanisms of reciprocal rejection and rupture with their resulting therapeutic discontinuity.

4. That organization of the treating teams within the community be directed toward ending the deadlock caused by adherence to traditional modes.
5. That the teamwork allow specific and differentiated interventions while maintaining permanent bonds with a coherent therapeutic program.
6. That technical and administrative responsibility for the creation and daily operation of the whole range of care institutions rest with the group of psychiatrists in charge of the sector teams.

Links Between Child and Adult Departments

In France, administrative confines often fetter the continuity of psychiatric care. In the association, however, the functions of the child and adult departments are closely coordinated in the heart of the same organization. Under these conditions continuity of care is assured for chronically ill patients, there is unity of action in relation to the family, and diagnosis is facilitated during a crisis when action is necessary, e.g., when hospitalization or incarceration of a parent takes place.

Particularly where adolescents are concerned, action has been made easier. Adolescents still in school are treated in the child department, whereas young people who are working are dealt with in the adult department. The advantages of rapport between the departments is such that in the restructuring of the mental health centers, two specialized teams, one for children and the other for adults, will function within one administrative unit.

The division of tasks between the two departments is not always easy or automatic. In most cases, the families of children in treatment are treated in the department of child psychiatry, yet even those parents who are obviously psychotic or very neurotic often do not look for help in the adult department. Constant harmony between the two departments on all levels is therefore necessary. To this end, all cases, both difficult and minor, are discussed in a seminar that includes all professionals with a permanent nucleus of consultants.

Unity of Responsibility and Continuity of Care

Although the close working relationship between the two departments is considered a technique for assuring unity and continuity, the most important point is that the hospital should not be the center of action. The vital cores are the mental health centers, where the first contact, the first attempt at diagnosis, and the first decisions are made, except for urgent cases needing immediate hospitalization.

In each of the centers, geographically separated for the time being, eight teams of specialists for children and eight teams for adults, somewhat varying in composition, are responsible for a defined territory within the arrondissement. Teams in the child department include a psychiatrist, social worker, psychologist, and technicians (psychoanalysts for psychotherapy and logopedics, i.e., specialized reeducators, for school problems, writing difficulties, and psychological problems). A team in the adult department generally includes a psychiatrist, social worker, psychoanalysts, specialists in rehabilitation, and nurses.

Each team has permanent responsibility for its patients, no matter where the care is being administered. Since the psychiatrists working full time in the adult department give half their time to the mental health center and the other half to an institution, permanent supervision is assured. In addition, since there are no social workers in the institutions, continuity of psychosocial work with the families (social casework) is essential.

To assure that the teams are kept up to date, a sheet is sent daily to each, listing the availability of free places in the institutions. In addition, the location of each patient is defined clearly in his record, where each change is scrupulously indicated. Although some institutions make visiting difficult, each team regularly visits its hospitalized patients.

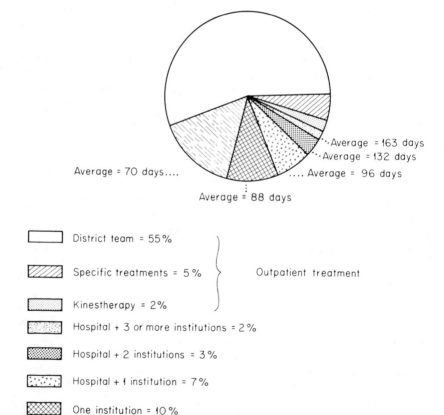

Fig. 4-2. Average yearly use of different types of therapy, 1965–1971.

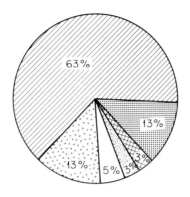

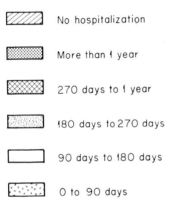

No hospitalization

More than 1 year

270 days to 1 year

180 days to 270 days

90 days to 180 days

0 to 90 days

Fig. 4-3. Distribution of patients according to accumulated hospitalization time, 1965–1971.

While the principles of continuous care and responsibility are simple, certain realities complicate the situation. First, there is the risk that the team, burdened with many responsibilities, will lean too heavily on the hospital, and we find once again the traditional dichotomy between hospital care and outpatient care. A second problem arises when patients and their families tend to become attached to the hospital, which gives them a feeling of security and reinforces the team's tendency to abandon the case.

We have come to the conclusion that a district psychiatric service should group its technical units in one place. We now plan to unite the two mental health centers in the same building to minimize the risk of losing sight of common objectives by separating the professionals into small, dispersed groups.

Operational studies by the association have shown, for the group of patients whatever their diagnosis, the accomplishments both of therapeutic activities and of the use of institutions (hospital and institutions outside the hospital). A 6-year study (1965–1971) shows annual averages concerning the use of different kinds of treatment (Figs. 4-2 and 4-3).

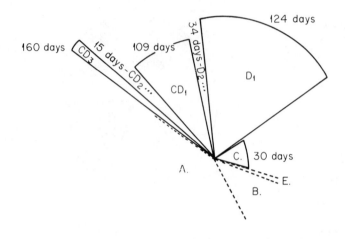

C = Hospital
D_1 = One institution
D_2 = Two institutions
CD_1 = Hospital + one institution
CD_2 = Hospital + two institutions
CD_3 = Hospital + three or more institutions

A = District team
B = Specific treatments } Outpatient treatment
E = Kinestherapy

Fig. 4-4.   Average yearly use of therapeutic facilities by neurotic patients, 1965–1971.

Examination of the use of therapeutic facilities by psychotic and neurotic patients shows that it is not only the types of patients habitually considered the most difficult who consume the most institutional time (Figs. 4-4 and 4-5). This and other research suggests that treatment of neurotics is particularly ineffective, practically speaking, in public services where the psychotherapeutic facilities are insufficient or where the professional's time is occupied entirely by psychotics, who are cared for entirely by the public services. In this situation, neurotics are examined and treated too late, often when depression is dominant and psychotherapy has little chance of being helpful. The institutions then risk being overloaded with neurotic patients.

These findings lead us to believe that our community service should deal more specifically with problems of neurosis. It is probably not necessary for neurotics to be subjected to the long diagnostic procedure usually required by the teams. The association is proposing creation of a service for psychoanalytic and

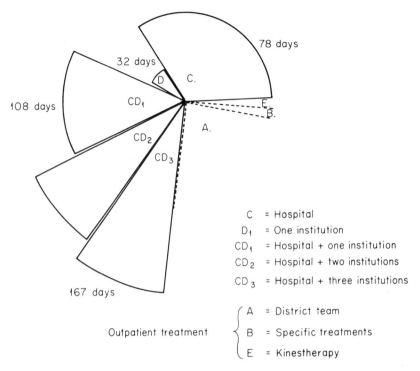

Fig. 4-5. Average yearly use of therapeutic facilities by psychotic patients, 1965–1971.

psychotherapeutic care in the hope that the patients will take the initiative of contacting a psychoanalyst or psychotherapist when the suggestion has been made to them. This therapeutic approach is somewhat different from current practice. It assumes that the case will be handled by a specialized and responsible team that will maintain close contact with all the services of the association.

Psychoanalytic Orientation of Services

Services in this district are largely oriented to psychoanalytic theory and technique. In both the child and adult departments, psychoanalysts are responsible for psychotherapy—psychoanalysis, psychoanalytic psychotherapy, group psychotherapy, and analytic psychodrama. Some of the psychiatrists, especially in the child department, have been psychoanalysts for a long time and are teaching in psychoanalytic institutes.

This predominance of psychoanalytic thought explains certain peculiarities, particularly in the child department. We utilize standardized diagnoses based on a classification which tries to describe each case in terms of psychoanalytic dynamics. In this situation, immediate observations are not considered essential. For example, the problems of learning to write (dyslexia, etc.) are often only the most visible manifestations of basic problems which are intensified by family and school intolerance; they are in fact related to much deeper emotional problems for which specific modalities of psychotherapy must be used.

When young children have not neutralized their sexual and aggressive impulses and lack proper development of symbolic thought and communication, they are threatened by profound disorganization leading to emotional or characterological difficulties. For those whom we consider "prepsychotic," psychoanalytic therapy can be of great importance.

The analysts' time, necessarily limited, is thus utilized for conceptual guidance. In the adult department the psychoanalysts work under analogous conditions, but the amount of patient psychotherapy undertaken is still small. Psychoanalytic theory enters on the level of initial and final evaluations, while the psychiatrists-psychoanalysts also try to improve object relationships in the institutions by using the perspectives of transference and countertransference.

Maintaining this effort under the exigencies of daily life on diverse services is not always easy. The psychoanalysts are not always prepared to take on these responsibilities and their reluctance is obvious when they try to correlate the observed facts with institutional and therapeutic practice. Some think there is a real incompatibility between the psychiatric function and psychoanalytic understanding.

We have been able to observe interactions closely in the 13th arrondissement. After a phase of goodwill, the psychoanalyst tends to withdraw from daily responsibilities in order to care for certain privileged patients in his office. Nonetheless, he remains an attractive model to others, who may try to imitate him, frequently substituting the administration of care for interpretations. Although there is always the risk that the nonpsychoanalyst will involve himself in interpersonal relations without fully considering his own involvement, we nevertheless believe that the psychoanalytical exposure is for us a practical tactic as well as an intellectual tool.

For example, in teamwork the psychoanalyst seems to us more open to understanding interpersonal difficulties. In his relations with the patient even outside psychotherapy, we believe he is capable of listening, of identifying to a reasonable degree, and of better controlling the massive countertransference relations set off by psychotics. Inside the institutions, he responds to the needs of groups of patients and their families.

The facts of psychiatric teamwork are sufficiently well known so that we need not discuss them here. It is sufficient to say that if he accepts working without the couch, the psychoanalyst is probably the best prepared to satisfy these necessities more by what he is than by what he says or interprets. He is perhaps better prepared than others to work efficiently in the community.

Work *in* and *for* the Community

The term "district psychiatry" has a slightly military sound in France. "Community psychiatry" is the term used in Anglo-Saxon countries. But in the 13th arrondissement we prefer to speak of "psychiatric work *in* the community."

The activities which use the institutions and the people of the community, we call "mediation." Our intermediaries in the community are the specialized agencies, and it is on these that we concentrate our efforts. (First, we must emphasize that using well-meaning but nonprofessional personnel is badly accepted in France. The labor unions fear that specialists will be employed less frequently because of an abundance of poorly prepared volunteers in all fields.)

The association's first mediation was with the public schools in the hope of averting the need for psychiatric help stemming from scholastic difficulties. At the beginning of our project we sent specialists trained in specific problems, particularly dyslexia, into the schools. We treated children who needed reeducation but whose parents could not collaborate with us, either because of lack of money or because of an incapacity to go along with an effort of this kind. Our presence in the schools has provided fruitful contacts with teachers and with the school authorities whom we can sensitize to the difficulties of child development. It was thus that we began our long history as consultants to the responsible figures in national education. One result is the existence of specialized agencies in France for "unadapted" children.

In the 13th arrondissement we were fortunate that all the special classes in the schools were created in consultation with us: Special classes for children who adapt badly to school life, classes which encourage discouraged children to make an effort (comparable to rehabilitation workshops for adults and provided for children discharged from psychiatric hospitals). Throughout this work, we were able to approach teachers, individually or in groups, to discuss common problems. We found older teachers mired in a routine out of which they will never move; the younger ones came to understand certain aspects of scholastic failure which they had formerly attributed to lack of will or to laziness. Their sensitivity to affective problems, their understanding of the various aspects of their relations with their students and their students' parents are very useful on condition that they accept their own roles and avoid experiments in laissez faire and nondirectiveness, a tendency which has required vigilance on our part.

For more than 10 years we have conducted a longitudinal study of two classes, begun when this group of children entered public school. From this study, we formulated ideas on the evolution of certain symptoms, on the future of patient pathology, and on the importance of the family milieu in relation to the future of these problems. The inadequacy of family support and its cultural consequences emerged as an essential element leading to mental deficiency.

The association has also collaborated with centers for maternal and infantile protection (well-baby clinics), and their adjunct prenursery schools. In France, it is difficult to remain a consultant without acting directly. Pediatricians are still not prepared (except with common sense) to play the role of psychologist. At the beginning of our work, it was important to point out to them that although they are knowledgeable about nursing and other interactions of young children and their mothers, they need not try to provide a psychiatric consultation. Our efforts were directed toward helping to define the specific role of the pediatrician with regard to preventive measures in the service of mental health.

Both in the schools and at the nursing centers, the personnel little by little acquired new knowledge, aided by our professionals, particularly the psychologists. Thus, we decided in time to become less active, either to withdraw or to act as specialized consultants. This changing role appears to us very important for the success of community psychiatry in all aspects of its mediate action.

Specialized Services for the Aged

We proceeded in much the same way in our development of specialized services for the aged. In France the help given to the elderly is often badly coordinated. Rapid modifications in our society and accelerated urbanization have intensified the nuclear character of the family, contributing to the suppression and isolation of the aged. Their lack of social life and medical care is responsible for the increasing number of aged persons admitted to psychiatric hospitals, as well as for the large percentage of deaths during the period of hospitalization.

Recognizing this problem, we founded a gerontopsychiatric service in our association. Through systematic interviews we determined the needs of the elderly. In cooperation with other institutions already involved in providing health and leisure-time services for the aged, we then organized an association of gerontology in the 13th arrondissement. Although it is autonomous, several of our psychiatrists collaborate with it. As part of this service two day centers and two leisure clubs for the aged have been opened. A home care division which collaborates with the hospital services that specialize in gerontology, devotes itself entirely to administering somatic medical care. These services have succeeded in limiting the need for psychiatry among the elderly.

Table 4-1 shows the results of our efforts. On December 31, 1970 the percen-

Table 4-1
Results of Gerontopsychiatric Service, December 31, 1970

	13th Arrondissement		Other Regions	
	Men	Women	Men	Women
Patients over 65 in psychiatric hospitals, as percent of all patients	10.52	39.24	12.79	37.49
Patients over 65 deceased in psychiatric hospitals, as percent of patients over 65 admitted	9.09	2.15	30.37	37.55
Patients over 65 deceased in psychiatric hospitals, as percent of patients over 65 released	10.00	2.22	37.00	55.48

tage of patients in the psychiatric district service of the 13th arrondissement was almost identical to the percentage for all of the psychiatric hospitals in the region of Paris. However, note the percentages concerning death compared with total admissions and with total releases. The results, we believe, are linked to our policy of short-term hospitalization, both in the specialized services of the general hospital and in the psychiatric hospital, and by our taking care of patients at home as well as in day-care centers.

Senility is still treated as another mental illness, and the open-door policy is applied to the senile at the hospital. This policy, as well as other policies of community psychiatry, involves the risk of some failure. However, we must convince the public authorities that these risks must be taken. We have tried to educate the public and particularly those people who are politically, administratively, or technically responsible. This we must do either on an individual level in specific cases, or in consultations on general problems, such as adolescent suicide, the use of drugs, and so on. In Anglo-Saxon countries, one can hope for positive action from politically responsible people; in France one must rather have faith in the effects of dialogue with a variety of specialists.

Certain of these difficulties are not unique to our services. Psychiatrists sin by their ignorance of certain realities of family life. On the other hand, specialized agencies tend either to ask too much of psychiatrists, in order to relieve themselves of unbearable pressures in particularly difficult cases, or to not consult psychiatrists at all, for many different reasons. Also, our contact with family doctors was difficult for some time, possibly because they feared that a district service would menace private medicine and the freedom to choose one's doctor.

Care for Families

Two of our services have had a deep effect on the families in our district. One is a parents' film club that meets to view dramatizations of interpersonal problems, which are then discussed with the assistance of a discussion leader sent by our service. The other is home care. An assigned team works with the families of patients who can be helped without being hospitalized. This form of psychotherapy includes the entire family group, and whenever possible, families living in the same building and neighborhood as well. In addition, this service runs a discussion group at the center for patients' families and other families to discuss inter- and intrafamily problems.

In both the adult and child departments, certain families are found to adjust badly to our psychiatric approach. Frequently we approach them through their children who present problems of language, lack of intellectual aptitude as shown through psychological testing, or tendencies toward evolving psychopathic aspects of personality. We find we are dealing with specific problems which emanate from the parents, who are often alcoholic or present other unstable aspects of behavior. These families are grouped in specific neighborhoods and are well known to social and psychiatric services.

Their recourse to psychiatric help stems from despair, and help is needed for reasons which these families are incapable of understanding. What does difficulty in learning to write signify for some of these mothers? Inversely, the psychiatric teams are not particularly knowledgeable about these families, who, in France at least, are not defined by economic misery: Their resources are no lower than those of most workers' families. The use of their resources, however, is special. The nature of their economic behavior seems to indicate that they need the excitement of being in debt, much like gamblers. Sudden and unplanned expenses, awkward and unlimited use of credit, a need for periodic sumptious feasts and extravagant unplanned-for gifts for the children are some of the manifestations of their personalities.

The husbands are unstable in their work, frequently gamblers or alcoholics. The women, tired by numerous pregnancies, tend to be depressive. Their inappropriate use of public services permits them often to get rid of their children by placing them here and there. Absence of consistent care and its resulting separations undoubtedly are the genesis of the children's complicated and badly defined symptoms, dominated by instability, intellectual and cultural retardation, and acting out. There is no one community service equipped, materially or intellectually, to satisfy the specific needs of these families. Social services limit themselves to providing material help or pretending to help on the educational level; the psychiatric services do not know how to form a stable and understanding relationship with these families. Their numerous problems require concerted effort on the part of all the social agencies which tend to deal with them in a disorganized way.

We have attempted to coordinate the efforts of all social agencies. For example, there is a small area of the 13th arrondissement where the children are almost all subnormal, where the adolescents form fighting gangs and use drugs, and where the families receive aid from a number of different agencies. We took the initiative to bring together representatives of the services involved for a seminar dealing with these cases. Among the many people who attended were social workers, club leaders, the youth leaders of preventive services for adolescents belonging to gangs, policemen, teachers, and of course, members of the psychiatric team for the district. In addition to better defining the specific nature of these families with multiple problems, we try to integrate the efforts undertaken and to find the best medium for dealing adequately with each problem.

The "hospitalization at home" service tries to be open to original ways of responding to ambiguously formulated demands. In the child department, an "evening intensive care unit" is provided for those still in school who are totally unmotivated intellectually. These children are received as a group after school, a dangerous time for them because of the absence of a welcoming family structure at home. At the center they can feel the interest of adults and are encouraged to substitute verbal communication for physical violence. Although these are not regular psychotherapeutic sessions, psychonalysts are present with the children and intervene directly during difficult moments of conflict, without an elaboration of the transference situation.

These children's teachers too are invited to the center, to talk about their pupils. Talents initially difficult to recognize are frequently brought to light. Parents are included in these pinpointed interventions in an effort to create a coherent discourse that will satisfy objective and subjective needs in interpersonal relations. Two years of this experiment appear to confirm that positive results can be accomplished in this area.

In the case of the problem families, we believe it best to avoid all preconceived ideas; instead, opinion should be based as closely as possible on the real lives of these families. Our focus, therefore, is on "naturalistic observation." Daily action in the community demands both creativity and rigor of investigation, which permit better control of the tasks undertaken and better use of personnel.

Research and Teaching

This last example and others to which we have alluded, such as the longitudinal studies conducted by the child department, remind us that controlled systematic studies lead naturally to research. Aside from those controlled by perspectives of our operations or related to our clinics, it seems to us useful to employ epidemiological and operational tools.

With the means at our disposal, it is difficult to do epidemilogical research dealing, for example, with the frequency of psychiatric morbidity in our population. But we try to compare the group with subgroups of the nonconsulting population, even if these patients are not representative samples.

For each patient in the two departments, we keep up to date an admission paper and a release paper. The former gives information on the patient's civil, social, economic, and cultural situation; financial status; diagnosis; prognosis; and treatment envisaged upon admission. The release paper includes a description of the circumstances at termination of care, the diagnosis and prognosis, conditions that surrounded application for care, and the condition of the patient upon release.

Obviously, utilizing these statistics, which are reviewed annually, demands agreement concerning the diagnostic options. This led us to propose that the diagnoses be recorded; some exercises in diagnosis may be done with the help of videotape.

At the same time, a study of socioeconomic characteristics of the population we have surveyed led to comparative researches based on certain given demographics of the 13th arrondissement. We soon observed, however, that these statistical studies were insufficient and that more extensive studies of certain characteristics of this population should be undertaken. Thus, a comparative study was made between the 13th and another district on the reaction of the community to mental illness.

In the 13th, our service is generally well known and is accepted as the place to go for the care of mental illness, just as one turns to other institutions during physical illness. Our association is felt to be protective of the family and of the society. In the other, less well-staffed arrondissement, the mentally ill person is still viewed as a strange and dangerous individual.

This example demonstrates how a series of researches develops from each inquiry and explains why we have not formed an autonomous research unit. As clinicians take on institutional responsibilities, we insist that the researchers keep touch with daily reality by being involved in the clinical and technical activities.

Through our psychiatric services, we have become conscious of the need for research concerning the specialists' time which is absorbed in daily tasks. Often overall demands and needs are lost sight of. For example, passivity regarding the waiting list for consultation or for the various therapies led to an aggravation of the causes for it. Statistical facts must be brought to the attention of the teams, since they reflect not only the activity of the service, but also the problems within it.

Experience has shown that when we discuss these problems the cohesion of the teams is assured. The usefulness to us of this kind of information has increased. In essence, this is a form of in-service teaching that can be envisioned within a service of this kind. In addition, those of us working with the universities carry further responsibilities in the teaching of community psychiatry.

CONCLUDING OBSERVATIONS

In describing certain aspects of community psychiatric services in the 13th arrondissement, we have not tried to hide some difficulties which have appeared over the years and which, perhaps, are specific, at least in part, to the situation in France.

Because the services in our district are more complete and more diversified than those of many other district psychiatric services, our expenses are said to be high. However, total expenditures in 1970 for the department of general psychiatry (adult) remain less per patient than would be spent in a comparable community which uses 3 psychiatric beds per 1000 inhabitants.

Our services, with a balance of therapeutic and preventive work, can be put under scrutiny on several other counts: Obstruction of the teams when the number of patients becomes too large to allow harmonious distribution of each member's time (even a minor overload can radically change the working conditions), and problems with elderly sick people who come to the service after having spent so much time in institutions that their pathology has become chronic. These situations, among others, can dangerously weaken our service, which is totally and without question dedicated to serving the psychiatric needs of the people.

While we must convince the authorities that we do not spend more money per subject treated than other kinds of psychiatric services, we must also keep alive our conception of psychiatry and resist becoming watered down into a social, charitable or political activity.

A district psychiatric service, we feel, should be responsive to the particular psychiatric needs of its community. Its specific functions are defined in terms of other institutions and by its daily actions. It seeks to allow the mentally ill, whom the community wants to expel, to continue living harmoniously within the community without losing the benefit of psychiatric help, whether in the hands of psychiatrists, the psychiatric services, or the non-psychiatric services.

Continual follow-up of our efforts and the reflections which they require are, in any case, indispensable to avoid the pitfalls of participating in the regressive organization of psychiatric services which forced those people, incapable of living in our demanding society because of their mental illness, to live in exile. Our apparatus could be called a tool of readaptation put to the service of a society which tends to reject all of its deviants.

PART II

Current Special Problems and Special Services in Community Mental Health

Nathan Sloate

5
Old Age

THE NEED

The existing imbalance between the mental health needs of the elderly and the availability of resources to serve them is receiving increased public exposure. The President's Task Force on the Aging (1970) expressed its concern regarding "the use of State mental hospitals as custodial facilities for large numbers of chronically ill or disabled older persons who are not in need of active psychiatric care because alternative living arrangements with psychiatric consultation or support do not exist."[1]

The Senate Special Committee on Aging, in anticipation of the White House Conference on Aging in 1971, issued a report entitled "Mental Health Care and the Elderly: Shortcomings in Public Policy," which referred to the "widespread confusions and contradictions in public health policy on mental health of the elderly [which] are causing heavy economic, social and psychological costs among older Americans and their offspring."[2] These costs are paid by some elderly misplaced in institutions when they could—with appropriate services—return to the community. Others pay that cost by remaining in their own homes, "in confusion or despair, denied access to services which help others but not them."[2]

The Group for the Advancement of Psychiatry, in its publication *Toward a Public Policy on Mental Health Care of the Elderly*, stated that "the elderly suffer disproportionately from our non-system of non-care, characterized by insufficient financing for both health and sickness and by fragmented delivery of services."[3]

The Special Concerns Session on Mental Health Care Strategies and Aging of the White House Conference recommended the establishment of a presidential commission on mental illness and the elderly and proposed that there be recognition and support of the individual's right to care and treatment within the full range of mental health services, that adequately staffed and programmed comprehensive local mental health services be developed for the elderly, and that greater efforts be made to develop alternatives to institutional care.[4]

The most potent force for greater equity in resource allocation is the elderly themselves. Their membership in senior citizen organizations, now over 600,000, multiplied 10-fold during the last decade. The older citizen is no longer satisfied to be at the mercy of the service providers. He recognizes that one of the great losses of old age is that of choice. He would like to bargain with dignity in the marketplace and to bargain as freely as any other consumer. This he can do only when services are available and options are assured.

Psychopathology in general and depression in particular rise sharply with age. Suicide reaches its zenith in elderly white males. One National Institute of Mental Health study shows the following incidence of psychopathology by age per 100,000 population (Table 5-1).

Table 5-1
Incidence of Psychopathology, by Age

Age Range	New Cases per 100,000 Population
Under 15	2.3
25–34	76.3
35–54	93.0
Over 65	236.1

Source: Biometrics Branch, OPPE, NIMH

Because of physiological changes, physical handicaps, multiple losses through death and separation, sharply diminished availability of sexual gratification, loss of social and work status, diminished income or financial dependency, older persons may lose confidence in themselves, become isolated and lonely, feel worthless, useless, or depressed. They become more vulnerable. They need socialization, good health care, special housing arrangements, or assistance in maintaining themselves in their own homes—all elements on a continuum which includes mental health. Mental health program achievement depends on the maintenance of the interrelationships along the continuum.

But the facts point to an accumulation of untreated illness. Resources are scattered and often inappropriately used. This is particularly the case in congregate care facilities, which provide 85 percent of the mental health care received by the elderly. Today 1 million elderly are living in state mental hospitals and nursing homes throughout the country—many as involuntary guests of the taxpayer. At least 30 percent (300,000) of these persons are not primarily in need of the services these facilities can provide and would be better off in a different kind of environment.

The scarcity of community resources, including mental health services, limits the range of choice. Full use is not being made of family and community potential. Strengthening of the programs to realize this potential will lessen the pressure on more expensive institutional care, will permit the institutions to serve their remaining residents better, and will help correct an imbalance as damaging to society as to the elderly.

HISTORICAL PERSPECTIVE

This national exposure of the issue of adequate mental health care for the elderly and the growing agreement on the need to develop a wider range of choices for the older consumer climax a historical development that began to accelerate after World War II. At that time few options were available to the older person and his family. Community resources were sparse or nonexistent. Families faced with the necessity for supplementary assistance that would enable them to keep their older member at home, finding none, resorted to the state mental hospital. This led to a mushrooming demand for state hospital beds, with resultant overcrowding, increased danger of spread of infectious diseases, and harshly circumscribed treatment programs. Governor Warren of California, during this period observed that if the state hospital population continued its present rate of growth, a new 2000-bed state hospital would be needed every year in his state. To cope with this runaway situation, California intensified its return to communities of patients no longer needing hospital care through a more active program of augmenting community resources, careful placement, and follow-up. That program succeeded in ultimately reducing that state's hospital population from a high of over 32,000 to less than 10,000 in 1972. This achievement was the product of a policy that no person should be inappropriately admitted or detained in a state hospital. Its basic humanism along with a commitment to achieve measurable and beneficial results gained widespread public and legislative support.

Particularly helpful in the community relocation of patients were the emerging federal programs. Beginning with old-age assistance and old-age insurance—practically the only public resources available during the 1940s—programs began to respond to the more obvious needs for protective services, income, housing, health and mental health care. No longer was it so imperative to hospitalize a citizen because housing was not available. Nor was it so essential that the older person go to a mental hospital because adequate medical care was not available. With the advent of programs such as medicare, medicaid, aid to the partially and totally disabled, the growth in income benefits, and the passage of the National Mental Health Act which opened the way for comprehensive community mental health services, the pressure for state hospital admissions and retentions began to diminish. Services became more accessible and acceptable. State hospitals no longer served as all things to all people.

Community-based mental health facilities more than doubled from 1960 to

1968, increasing from 22 to 32 percent of all psychiatric facilities during this period. Whereas in 1955 patients under care in mental hospitals were 2.5 times the number treated in outpatient psychiatric services, by 1968 that balance had shifted so that half a million more patients were served in community facilities than in hospitals.

FUNDING LIMITATIONS

But the patterns of delivery of services responding to these developments are severely limited and often determined by the source of their financing. A visit to a residential care center for the elderly, which was developing a day-care program as an addition to its 24-hour-care program, revealed that it was easier to obtain the more expensive funding for full-time residential care than for the day-care program because of the restrictions in medicare and medicaid, although by staff judgment easily 30 percent of the full-time residents would have been better served in the day-care program.

Table 5-2 provides a summary of estimated medicare and medicaid expenditures for health and psychiatric services for persons aged 65 and over for fiscal years 1967–69. It is clear that not only were expenditures for mental health services modest compared with the total expenditures but they decreased from 4.5 percent in 1967 to 3.7 percent in 1969. Even of this meager share, the proportion of expenditures for other than hospital care was negligible.

The $250 annual total limitation under medicare for outpatient mental health services is a clear example of how hospitalization is encouraged for services that might better be provided on an outpatient basis. This limitation does not apply when the professional renders medical or psychiatric care to a mentally ill beneficiary who is an inpatient, regardless of whether the patient's 150 days of inpatient hospital services in a benefit period or the 190 days inpatient psychiatric hospitalization lifetime limit have expired.

The Group for the Advancement of Psychiatry notes that the limitation "not only affords inadequate coverage but promotes hospitalization rather than care in the community, often contrary to sound psychiatric practice."[3] The President's Task Force on the Aging concurred on this point: "Medicare coverage of outpatient psychiatric treatment . . . is so limited that it discourages older persons from seeking help and encourages practitioners to hospitalize older persons who may not require hospitalization so that they can receive treatment."[1] The task force explicitly recommended "that the restrictions in Medicare coverage on outpatient psychiatric care be removed so that Medicare pays the same benefits for outpatient psychiatric treatment as it does for all other medical care."[1]

The President's Task Force on the Mentally Handicapped,[6] after considering the limitations on benefits for the mentally impaired, recommended that all provisions discriminating against the mentally disabled be removed from medicare and medicaid laws, regulations, and administration, and that the government devel-

Table 5-2

Estimated Medicare and Medicaid Reimbursements, All Services, and Psychiatric Services, Fiscal 1967–1969 (in millions, except percentages)

Program and Type of Service	1967 Total	1967 Psychiatric Amount	1967 Psychiatric Percent of Total	1968 Total	1968 Psychiatric Amount	1968 Psychiatric Percent of Total	1969 Total	1969 Psychiatric Amount	1969 Psychiatric Percent of Total
Total	$5,332	$241	4.5	$8,569	$330	3.8	$10,646	$400	3.7
Medicare	3,395	50	1.5	5,347	75	1.4	6,598	93	1.4
Hospital care	2,406	48	2.0	3,414	71	2.1	4,301	88	2.0
General hospitals	2,394	36	1.5	3,394	51	1.5	4,275	62	1.5
Psychiatric hospitals	12	12	100.0	20	20	100.0	26	26	100.0
Physicians' services	626	2	0.3	1,291	4	0.3	1,492	5	0.3
Other	363			642			805		
Medicaid	1,937	191	9.9	3,222	255	7.9	4,048	307	7.6
Hospital	830	191	23.0	1,300	255	19.6	1,529	307	20.0
Other	1,107			1,922			2,519		

Source: US Department of Health, Education, and Welfare: Research Report No 37. Financing Mental Health Care Under Medicare and Medicaid. Washington DC, GPO, 1971.

op and promote legislative and administrative measures to enhance the capacity of the service system.

The General Accounting Office recently blamed the lack of planning and underutilization of community treatment, including the "virtual neglect of preventive medicine," for rising federal health care costs. These costs jumped from $26 billion in 1960 to $75 billion in 1971, increasing the average cost of hospitalization from $32 a day in 1960 to $91 in 1971.

Thus we find our experts in agreement—but the exclusions and discriminations remain.

NEGATIVE ATTITUDES: CAUSE AND EFFECT

Research findings during the past decade suggest that functional mental impairment in older persons is as responsive to treatment as in others who are younger, and that apathy, isolation, and regressed behavior can be reduced by adequate assessment of the improvement potential and the specific modes of intervention. There is mounting evidence of the rehabilitation potential of the elderly by practitioners in the field. Yet somehow this has not been translated into practice.

Considerable research has dealt with negative attitudes that permeate the area of geriatrics. Both administrative and treatment staff inappropriately fear that the elderly are unresponsive and unrehabilitatable. Popular misconceptions about treatability often delay the seeking of help until a crisis develops. Students in general have negative attitudes toward working with older people. Lutz and Gaitz[7] studied the attitudes of psychiatrists toward the aged and aging by means of mail questionnaires to 435 psychiatrists. Only 40 percent responded. The questioners found strong prejudices among the psychiatrists against treating the aged.

One of the major factors causing society to turn away from the elderly has to do with the reality of death, which is associated with the older person, and our cultural denial of this reality. In a study of 348 elderly patients at a New York State mental hospital, Markson and Hand[8] concluded that mental hospitals are being used as an "easy out" for terminal patients. Elderly persons referred to the geriatric services of mental hospitals are from socioeconomically deprived, low education levels. Their low status leads to inappropriate hospitalization. This could be mitigated by diminishing the number of cursory psychiatric examinations and by using psychiatric screening programs. Public education was suggested to teach the public and professionals to understand the right of the elderly to die in the comfort of their homes with the emotional support of their families.

One of the most obvious obstacles to delivery of services to the elderly is the often detrimental and sometimes fatal effect of relocation into an institution. Kasl reviewed the literature on relocation stress and concluded:

Relocation and/or institutionalization will have adverse effects on the physical and psychological well being of the elderly if: (a) it increases the physical distance to friends, kin, and age peers, as well as to various services and facilities; (b) it interferes with their engaging in their usual leisure and social activities; (c) it represents a deterioration in the quality of their dwelling unit and their neighborhood and valued dimensions.[9]

These detrimental effects are preventable with careful casework service and psychological support.

Community agency resistance to the mentally impaired older person is manifested by reluctance to qualify for basic benefits possible candidates for institutional care. Even old-age assistance for patients leaving state mental hospitals was once opposed by welfare departments, who did not see these applicants as their responsibility.

A POSITIVE APPROACH

Treatment goals are often different for the elderly than for the young. They do not always imply recovery. Slowing the progress of the disease may be called for. Return to productivity is not so applicable. Traditional therapies, including psychotherapy, are as useful for the elderly as for the younger patients. One study concluded that the group therapy approach is very successful with the elderly, as long as the patients are receptive to social interaction and have been selected and prepared for entry into a group program. Wolk and Goldfarb[10] studied the response to 1 year of group psychotherapy in 26 aged recent admissions compared with 24 long-term mental hospital patients. "In both long-term patients and new admissions in old age, group psychotherapy seems to ameliorate depression, facilitate good interpersonal relations and improve self concept." It was noted that decreases in anxiety, depression, and improvement in interpersonal relations can be achieved even when organic brain syndrome is present. Work and Goldfarb concluded: "Group psychotherapy appears to be universally helpful but benefits aged schizophrenics more than aged persons with chronic brain syndrome who are first admitted to mental hospitals late in life."

Because older persons must accept some degree of dependency on others, their therapy may focus on the reduction of the fear, anger, and antisocial behavior precipitated by such dependency. This is sometimes overlooked in our eagerness to respond to the broader needs of the elderly. Meeting these broader needs is sometimes easier than helping patients overcome their regression, anger, and passivity. The need in almost every patient for support, encouragement, guidance, and at times, psychotherapy should be of concern to the therapist.

In her classic study on aging and mental disorders in San Francisco in 1967, Lowenthal[11] made the following recommendations for practice:

1. Because physical illness parallels psychiatric illness in old age, their treatments should be available at the same time.
2. Acute organic brain syndrome is important to diagnose because it is often treatable.
3. For those who must care for themselves in the community, inability to do so frequently precipitates psychiatric hospitalization.

4. Psychiatric illnesses are associated with multiple deprivations. Prevention may be achieved by overcoming these.
5. Institutional admissions often represent the breakdown of previous long-term care provided by the families.
6. Community mental health services are needed but would require vigorous out-reach for older persons, particularly the poor, because of these persons' fear of such institutions.

Some measure of service deficiency to the elderly is suggested by Table 5-3 which shows the percent distribution of patient care episodes for community-based care in 1969. The elderly are drastically underrepresented in relation to their proportion in the population and even more importantly in relation to the higher incidence of psychopathology known to exist within this age group. A more precise breakdown of admission patterns to outpatient care is given in Table 5-4. It shows the marked contrast in the proportion of admissions in the 65-plus group as compared with the younger service recipients.

The community mental health center program was authorized by Congress in 1963 to better respond to the national need for mental health services available to people where they live. Centers were expected to provide at least five essential elements of service to a given geographical area ranging in population from 75,000 to 200,000:

1. 24-Hour inpatient services
2. Outpatient services
3   Partial hospitalization
4. Emergency services
5. Consultation and education

Recommended for fully comprehensive care, but not mandated, were

6. Rehabilitation services
7. Training
8. Research and evaluation
9. Diagnostic services
10. Precare and aftercare

The comprehensive program of the centers includes special services for such groups as the elderly. In practice these have been minimal.

Data on characteristics of patients using these centers are limited owing to the newness of the program. The most recent statistics available are for 1969. Table 5-5 shows the percent distribution of patient care episodes for community mental health centers in 1969. These constitute but a fraction of the 505 centers that were approved for 1973. Table 5-6 shows the number of patient care episodes in community mental health centers for the same year.

Should present trends of mental health service continue through 1980, it is projected that 80 percent of the elderly in need will never be served. Table 5-7 estimates the number and percent of persons needing and receiving psychiatric ser-

Table 5-3

Percent Distribution of Patient Care Episodes for Community-based Care, 1969

Mode	Numbers		Age (%)		Mode (%)	
	All Ages	Elderly	Nonelderly	Elderly	All Ages	Elderly
Community-based care	1,972,083	47,178	97.6	2.4		
Outpatient psychiatric service	1,894,460	45,315	97.6	2.4	100	100
Federally funded CMHC	291,148	8,152	97.2	2.8	15	18
VA outpatient	35,547	1,105	96.9	3.1	1.9	2.4
Other outpatient	1,567,765	36,058	97.7	2.3	82.8	79.6
Day treatment service	77,631	1,863	97.6	2.4	100	100
CMHC	16,949	407	97.6	2.4	21	21.8
Other	60,682	1,456	97.6	2.4	78.2	78.2

Source: Biometry Branch, OPPE, NIMH

Table 5-4

Age at Admission to Outpatient Psychiatric Care, 1969

	Total	<18	18–24	25–34	35–44	45–64	65+
Number	880,762	261,823	143,596	178,352	136,357	139,983	20,651
Rate per 100,000	441.1	370.2	671.9	746.4	594.8	338.9	106.1
Percent	100	29.7	16.3	20.2	15.5	15.9	2.4

Source: Biometry Branch, OPPE, NIMH

Table 5-5

Percent Distribution of Patient Care Episodes for CMHCs, 1969

		Age		
Facility	Percent	18	18–64	65+
Inpatient				
All facilities	100	6.3	78.0	15.7
CMHC	100	7.5	84.9	7.6
Outpatient				
All facilities	100	28.6	69.0	2.4
CMHC	100	26.2	71.0	2.8
Day treatment				
All facilities	100	11.4	86.2	2.4
CMHC	100	11.4	86.2	2.4

Source: Biometry Branch, OPPE, NIMH

Table 5-6

Number of Patient Care Episodes in CMHCs, 1969

	Age		
Facility	Under 65	65+	Total
Inpatient	60,060	4,940	65,000
Outpatient	282,996	8,152	291,148
Day care	10,542	407	16,949
Total	353,598	13,499	373,097

Source: Biometry Branch, OPPE, NIMH

Table 5-7
Estimated Number and Percent of Persons Needing, Receiving, and Not Receiving
Psychiatric Services (Assuming 10 Percent of Population in Need of Services) and Based
on Assumption of Continued Change in Use Rates of Services, All Ages and
65 Years and Over, United States, 1975 and 1980

	1975 (1955–1968 Use Rate Continues)		1980 (1955–1968 Use Rate Continues)	
	Number	*Percent*	*Number*	*Percent*
All ages				
Needing services	21,559,000		22,751,000	
Receiving services	3,636,000	16.9	4,337,000	19.1
Not receiving services	17,923,000	83.1	18,414,000	80.9
Elderly only				
Needing services	2,150,000		2,349,000	
Receiving services	411,000	19.1	490,000	20.9
Not receiving services	1,739,000	80.9	1,859,000	79.1

Source: Biometry Branch, OPPE, NIMH

vices in 1975 and 1980, based on a need for services by 10 percent of the population and assuming continued change in use rates of services.

The achievement of a comprehensive mental health program for the elderly
is linked to an active effort in training. Numbers and kinds of personnel serving
the old are a prerequisite for an adequate and successful service outcome. These
cadres must be suited to the needs of the aged. Compared with the vast need for
home health aides, for example, but a small fraction is available and equipped.

Table 5-8 estimates the need for and availability of professional services in
mental health for 1975 and 1980. Since the elderly are included among those needing the services, we can assume that the estimated manpower shortages will apply
to them as well.

The changing directions in future service delivery provide opportunity and potential for a flexible array of training approaches, whether in the existing core disciplines or in new hybrids. Experimental and special education can identify more
effective ways of equipping man to better serve his fellow man. For example, expanded provision of institutional support in training settings could bring the novice
worker and elderly patients together to overcome the former's uncertainties and

Table 5-8

Need for and Availability of Professional Services in Mental Health

Discipline	1975			1980		
	Required	Expected	Difference	Required	Expected	Difference
Psychiatry*	86,235	30,300	56,235	91,004	38,700	52,304
Psychology†	86,235	30,000	56,235	91,004	44,800	46,204
Social work‡	86,235	25,400	60,835	91,004	36,600	54,404
Nursing§	86,235	35,900	50,333	91,004	51,300	39,704

*One or more years of psychiatric training.
†M.A. or Ph.D. with training in mental health field.
‡M.A. with training in mental health field.
§Some training in psychiatric nursing.
Source: Division of Manpower and Training Programs, NIMH

fears in dealing with the latter. The service needs might even suggest requirements for a worker with a different kind of personality, who can find his rewards in more modest therapeutic gains than the traditional ones sought by the core disciplines.

PROSPECTS

It has often been said that the measure of a society is how it treats its old. For a variety of reasons, our culture equates age with obsolescence and orders its priorities accordingly. Were our value system otherwise, three fourths of the elderly would not be so poor or so ill housed or so isolated. Nor would they need to be misplaced in mental hospitals during the remaining years of their lives. We must assume that the elderly receive in community benefits that which we want them to receive—no more. It is ironic indeed that, according to the findings of one study, they give to their chiddren, even in material things, more than they receive.

Without a value system that commits itself to the achievement of equity for the old, the future of these people is bleak indeed. Motivation and resolve are the necessary prerequisites for achieving goals and overcoming program obstacles. A social commitment is required. A reward system must be adopted that incorporates the benefits to all of society as well as the elderly.

We have seen some promising signs. Not only have the elderly become more forceful protagonists of their own interests, but refreshingly, their cause is joined by the young. It was the young who succeeded in focusing national attention on low standards of care in congregate care institutions and who are continuing to press for their reform.

A great step forward has been taken by the courts in decisions concerning right to treatment. In *Lake* v *Cameron*, Judge Bazelon, U.S. Court of Appeals, upheld the legal right to alternative community facilities. A patient who had previously been committed to St. Elizabeth's Hospital was found not to need its psychiatric services and the court ruled she should not be deprived of her liberty. The patient was without financial resources to obtain the appropriate community care. Said Judge Bazelon: "Deprivations of liberty solely because of dangers to the ill persons themselves should not go beyond what is necessaary for their protection. The court's duty to explore alternatives in such a case [as this] is related also to the obligation of the state to bear the burden of exploration of possible alternatives an indigent cannot bear."

The U.S. Senate Special Committee on Aging, the President's Task Force on the Mentally Handicapped, the White House Conference on the Aging, and the various professional and citizen groups have all raised their voices urging a better life for the elderly.

In its report, the Group for the Advancement of Psychiatry urged:

Those who are professionally concerned about the prospects for the mentally ill aged have a special obligation to speak out in their behalf, for that group is nearly voiceless within the pluralistic system of interests competing for national attention and funds. It is not enough to study and come to understand the problems and potentials of various mental health programs; in the competitive arena of politics one must contend for their implementation.[3]

Suitable mental health service models for the elderly need to be oriented to the need priorities of the elderly. Criteria for useful models include availability; acceptability, with measurable outcome providing for administrative accountability; feasibility, with high payoff in achieving targeted objectives and congruent with the demands of the consumers and the community. Good programs should involve their recipients along with related community service providers in developing and evaluating program policy and practice. Because of the particular requirements of the elderly, a strong element of outreach is indicated. Coordination in the delivery of service is essential at the service or consumer level, regardless of the separate purposes of the agencies that may be involved. There must be a critical mass of adequacy and quality of service.

These criteria are suggested by the more successful outcomes of our demonstration and practice. Perhaps no existing model would fully satisfy these standards. Yet the conviction is growing that without a comprehensive perspective our progress will be limited.

We have much to learn about how to improve our system of care. Many questions arise about more suitable patterns of care. Not much is known about our system of incentives that encourage those who serve the elderly. Treatment outcome is far from being fully understood. The impact of financing on patterns of service is not yet clear. Better methods of treating and managing chronic brain syndrome must be learned. How to bring about better motivation among mental health professionals calls for greater understanding.

Yet the application of that which we already know about mental health services for the elderly, if fully accepted and supported by program administrators, program providers, and the public, can help bring about a whole new era for our older Americans.

REFERENCES

1. Toward a Brighter Future for the Elderly. Report of the President's Task Force on the Aging. Washington, DC, GPO, 1970
2. Mental Health Care and the Elderly: Shortcomings in Public Policy. Report by U.S. Senate Special Committee on Aging. Washington, DC, GPO, 1971
3. Group for the Advancement of Psychiatry. Toward a Public Policy on Mental Health Care of the Elderly. New York, GAP, 1970
4. 1971 White House Conference on Aging. Report to the delegates from the conference sections and special concerns sessions. Washington, DC, GPO, 1971
5. Group for the Advancement of Psychiatry. The Aged and Community Mental Health: A Guide to Program Development. New York, GAP, 1971
6. Report of the President's Task Force on the Mentally Handicapped. Washington, DC, GPO, 1970
7. Lutz C, Gaitz CM: Psychiatrists' attitudes toward the aged and aging. Gerontologist 12(2):163–167, 1972
8. Markson EW, Hand J: Referral for death: Low status of the aged and referral for psychiatric hospitalization. Aging Hum Dev 1(3):261–272, 1970
9. Kasl SV: Physical and mental health effects of involuntary relocation and institutionalization on the elderly: A review. Am J Public Health 62:377–383, 1972
10. Wolk RL, Goldfarb AK: The response to group psychotherapy of aged recent admission compared with long-term mental hospital patients. Am J Psychiatry 10:1252–1256, 1967
11. Lowenthal MF: Aging and Mental Disorders in San Francisco. San Francisco, Jossey-Bass, 1967

Irving N. Berlin, M.D.

6
Childhood

Community mental health centers have promised a great deal, and only rarely have they been able to make good. Especially tragic has been the promise of treatment for children and families and provision of early intervention and prevention programs for children. Conceived as an alternative to poorly functioning and dehumanizing state hospitals, the centers' primary commitment was to adults in state hospitals or those who would be candidates for state hospitals. The motto, ''Keep the mentally ill adults in the community to enhance their recovery,'' became the primary and often the sole function.[1a] The community mental health center, conceived in a health model to prevent hospitalization and chronicity, operates as a mental illness center.

Once a community mental health center is accepted by a community as a viable resource for the mentally ill and emotionally disturbed, it is quickly overwhelmed by the most vocal and demanding members of the community—the troubled adults and their agency representatives. It has become clear in assessing the paucity of mental health services for children that, however well intentioned the professional staff, the clamor for services from adults, young and old, drowns out the cries of children for help.[1]

Age-old rationalizations are heard both from concerned adults in the community and from mental health professionals questioned about the need to help children. Children still have a chance; maybe the schools, juvenile courts, YM or YWCAs, will make a difference for disturbed children. Adults have nowhere to turn except the state hospital. Even youngsters who have failed to make it in school are presumed to have more resiliency, more promise of adaptation than the tormented adults disturbing their environment, who seem to be at the end of their rope.[1a] Besides, as one psychiatrist pointed out, adult psychotics do well on antipsychotic medication and require only minimal follow-up. Severely disturbed chil-

dren are often resistant to most medication and seem to require prolonged psychotherapeutic or psychoeducational work, and their parents need to be involved; these
are major time investments. Acting-out, delinquent youths are especially difficult
to handle and are exhausting to already overworked center staff. Thus for many
reasons children's troubles are invisible until children are physically big enough to
create problems for the community.[1b]

One of the major reasons given for non-existent or inadequate services for
children is the lack of trained personnel to work diagnostically and therapeutically
with children and their families. However, in recent years more well-trained mental health professionals experienced in work with children have joined community
mental health centers only to find that they are used almost exclusively to work
with adults.

SOME MODELS OF EFFECTIVE CHILDREN'S SERVICES

In Baltimore, Chicago, Philadelphia, and several other cities there are bright
spots where services to children have become a commitment of a mental health
center. Most surprising, these centers in the main have developed innovative patterns of service growing out of a basic philosophic posture that prevention and early intervention are the primary goals.

In the Woodlawn area of Chicago the community's demand that the mental
health center ensure that children succeed in school and do not drop out, especially
in the hazardous third grade, resulted in an innovative approach to helping teachers, students, and parents examine how children can be helped to learn in primary
grades.[2,3] Their class discussion method in the first 3 years of school had visible
impact not only in improving the learning of children but also in reducing the
number of children diagnosed by teachers as disturbed and disturbing. Treatment
services for children in this community had equal priority with services for adults.

In Philadelphia[4] and Baltimore[5] prevention-oriented child psychiatrists
conceived different routes to early intervention in children's problems.

In Philadelphia a family approach to children's problems resulted in training
of mental health professionals and paraprofessionals to work with families of children identified early as having trouble in school. These efforts to understand the
dynamics of a family that resulted in an identified disturbed child focused on altering family interaction so that all members of the family, in addition to the identified child, might learn to function differently both in the family and out. Helping
parents to become ego integrative models for their children and to enhance their
children's learning and thus lessen disruptive behavior had a positive effect on the
entire family.[6]

Out of these efforts came a gradual awareness of the variety of strengths and
coping capacities within these troubled families. A number of strategies for enhancing the existent coping mechanisms and using specific family strengths to deal
with current stress, both external and internal to the family, were taught and prac-

ticed. The para, or new, professional from the community who understood the life styles and could interact naturally with families was utilized. More paraprofessionals were trained to work with families. As the center came to accept the family as the unit for intervention, some carry-over to schools and courts occurred in families that were rarely worked with around the troubles of a student.[7,8]

Alternative strategies began to emerge—working with disturbed family members individually in addition to family sessions; dealing with the family as a subunit of a neighborhood where several families with similar troubles might learn together how families and individuals might function more effectively.

The impact of such family interventions on young and still not seriously troubled children was clearly preventive. The decision to concentrate on providing early intervention for young school children in trouble was a conscious one which needed to be balanced against community demand for relief from the antisocial, destructive behavior of adolescents and for aid for mentally ill adults.[8]

In Baltimore the hypotheses to be tested were that there were important checkpoints in the early school life of children which would identify those who needed help, and further that the schoolteacher and principal had to be active members of the child mental health team. Their role was not only diagnostic—learning to identify children in trouble or potentially in trouble, as in Bowers' study,[9] they were also a critical part of the treatment team. Educators' attitudes, behaviors, and expectations with regard to a troubled student could do much to help the latter—both in learning new behaviors and in academic achievement. Both areas were critical to the child's self-concept, sense of competence, and thus his mental health.[10]

An easy flow system from school to outpatient, day-care, and inpatient children's services was slowly evolved. One critical and difficult personnel problem was to work out how a team composed of teacher and mental health worker would follow a child from school into clinical service and back. Inherent in the success of the operation was the early and continuous use of mental health personnel in the classroom to carry out the evaluations and to involve teachers in the assessment of their students. As mental health professionals and teachers collaborated as equals, they began to use each others' professional expertise and personal sensitivities and capacities to reach children and to mutually work toward resolution of students' problems.

This unique relationship with one elementary school in a ghetto mental health center with a commitment to children provides some guidelines for other collaborations.[5]

In yet another setting, emphasis was on helping parents in the community learn how to make their concern about failure and dropping out by their elementary-school children felt by the school.[11] In this housing development in a ghetto, the center's mental health professionals were primarily consultants and resource persons, although their access to the schools (where they also consulted and thus understood school viewpoints as well) enhanced their capacity to consult more relevantly with parents. Through meetings with the most concerned parents, whose children were not learning, they developed a model of parent involvement in school. The basic thesis was that if parents attended regularly in the classrooms to observe and collect data about how teaching and learning were occurring in each classroom, they would be in a stronger position to make meaningful recommendations for change and to insist on change based on their firsthand knowledge of the situation. From other experiences it was presumed that the usual evasions and put-offs would be less effective if parents knew firsthand the school situation.

The first issue to be dealt with was how to get a number of parents into classrooms as observers. The suggestion was immediately vetoed by the principal. The parents then had no recourse but to approach the community board. In this community a citizen board composed of elderly women and men dealt with most community relations to the agencies of the city—the welfare, health, and police departments, and the schools. The younger citizens of the various housing projects in the area rarely involved themselves with the board unless an emergency occurred and some favor or pressure was needed to influence an agency serving the community. The parents were reluctant to approach the board. Some 10 years previously it had been militant in defense of the rights of blacks on welfare and black youths in trouble with the law, but in recent years had been complacent and reluctant to actively engage the power structure. Initial requests by a delegation of the parent group that the board lean on the administration brought vague promises but no action. Finally the parent group decided that all 18 parents would show up at the next meeting and confront the community board with their request, making it clear they would continue to push the board at every meeting until they were admitted to the classrooms in the school.

By the next week permission was granted. Simple evaluation sheets, designed with the consultant's help, indicated at 10-minute intervals what was being taught to whom, what children were not involved, what nonlearning or disruptive behavior was tolerated, and for how long. Thus in a few weeks' time, clear documentation of the learning occurring in each classroom was recorded.

There then occurred a struggle to get the community board to push the superintendent and school board to transfer out the principal and those teachers clearly not able or willing to work at teaching the children. Over time, with increased political action on the part of the parents (electing several parents to the community board, leaning on the black city councilman to support them), they were able to bring about these changes.

Having learned how to gather data in the elementary-school setting, parents began to help others learn to collect evidence about welfare runarounds, health department clinic delays and maltreatment, and teaching effectiveness at the junior-high-school level.

The mental health task undertaken was to facilitate the effectiveness of parents in community action as a way of enhancing the mental health of the children. There was no doubt that the involved parents also became more effective, and thus their mental health was enhanced.

THE HEALTH–MENTAL HEALTH MODEL: THE MULTIPURPOSE APPROACH

Yet another model that is evolving in a number of settings regards health care as unitary and not separate from mental health services. There are obvious advantages to a holistic system of care. Children are seen regularly and early in health clinics for immunizations and for eye, ear, and dental examinations. Trained and sensitive health care workers can assess developmental progress and raise questions about developmental delays, malnutrition, frequent illnesses, family complaints about a child's behavior, signs of maternal stress, etc. Families receiving decent health care in a dignified setting are less defensive about discussing family concerns and problems, and the public health nurse who visits for postnatal care is accepted as someone who can come into the home and render a helpful service. The nurse is a natural therapeutic intervener in family problems requiring validation and observation or development of a trusting relationship to permit accurate assessment. Indigenous paraprofessionals also provide a natural avenue of inquiry and home visiting ranging from follow-up on health problems to helping the family work toward recognizing a mental health problem and accepting help.

Perhaps most striking in the health centers I know best is how quickly families learn that coming in to talk with a familiar person about anything that stresses or concerns them is helpful. Thus crises and severe maladaptive behavior can be avoided. In one setting, the pediatrician's concern with helping families learn to deal with the stress caused by chronic illness in a child led to more frequent requests for help with the stresses surrounding a dying grandparent or drug abuse by an adolescent. It was also clear that parents who learned to handle the severe stress around a chronically ill child could be effective in helping other parents in the center with similar problems.[12-15]

Another general health care center was related to the population served by an elementary school. The required school examinations of these youngsters brought parents in with their health problems. The family health care spread through inquiries about parents and siblings by the workers responsible for disseminating the information through home visits. In this setting, school problems were frequently discussed with the workers. This family health care system in a mental health center developed a team of health and mental health care personnel who worked together, referred to each other, and began to work as cotherapists with parent and adolescent groups. In these teams the paraprofessionals called themselves not therapists, but "behavior changers."[16,17]

Inherent in most of these models are the problems which come from inadequate resources to deal with overwhelming difficulties. However, the difficult issues of determining priorities—who will be served and how—also may lead to innovative efforts to deal with mental health and health problems which permit more accurate assessment of need, methods of meeting needs, the cost and relative efficacy of various interventions in meeting needs, and the worth of prevention and early intervention strategies.[17a]

DEVELOPMENTALLY BASED COMMUNITY
MENTAL HEALTH CENTER ACTIVITIES

Focus on Prevention

A community mental health center committed to a public health prevention model must concern itself with prevention of retardation and organic brain damage due to malnutrition both of mothers during pregnancy and of infants during the first few years of life. In this context the mental health center needs to be closely linked to welfare and health organizations to support vitamin and protein supplements to pregnant mothers and infants. Both health care systems need to focus on using neighborhood health workers to get pregnant women in for prenatal care and to plan for good care during delivery.[18-21]

Epidemiological Data

Epidemiological studies reveal that many mental health problems are more prevalent among poor and minorities. Malnutrition, prematurity and birth trauma to infants, and learning problems are more frequent in these populations. Mental illness in general and delinquency are also more frequent among poor and minorities.[18,20,22-28] Maternal depression and early mother-child alienation are found in all socioeconomic classes, but with more frequency among the poor. The same is true of child abuse, neglect, and failure to thrive.[13,29-31] Thus prevention and early intervention are critical to the efforts to deal with mental illness in the poor and minority populations.[32]

Research also indicates that maternal depression, usually prior to and during the first year of the child's life, is potentially a serious deterrent to the child's capacity to form attachments to mother and to form subsequent trusting relationships. Thus the degree of maternal depression and estrangement from the child may determine the degree of disturbance, from infantile psychoses to inhibition of curiosity and capacity to learn easily.[13,33-35]

CASE EXAMPLE

A 2-year-old child was referred to us by his pediatrician after he was hospitalized for pneumonia. In the hospital this child interacted very little with nurses. He protested not at all when given intravenous medication, and smiled only rarely as he related to one nurse. There was little of the usual 2-year-old curiosity. Though he said a few words to his mother, his speech was confined to a few verbs with staff. His immobile face concerned the pediatrician, who requested psychiatric consultation.

The child psychiatrist found it difficult to relate to the child and convinced the mother that an evaluation was in order when the latter described the baby's day as consisting mostly of sitting and rocking to music or putting a favorite pair of mother's shoes in and out of the shoe box. The mother recognized how limited his speech, motor, and social development was in comparison with that of an older sibling at the same age.

The mother had been ill with chronic ulcerative colitis during the pregnancy and birth. The father was away in the service during most of the boy's first year and the mother's colitis remained severe. The mother described serious depression and a feeling of relief that her baby was so "good," slept well, ate well, and lay in his crib not demanding attention, which she had to center on her active and demanding older child.

Although this boy looked autistic, he changed rapidly as we helped the mother to work out a program of stimulation. Mostly she talked, sang, and read to him, and played a variety of contact games in which both physical touch and muscular freedom and control were emphasized. In hide-and-seek, he ran away from her, and when she caught him, she threw him in the air and hugged him. It became a favorite game. In about 4 months he lost all his autistic symptoms, and although he was fearful of agemates, he smiled warmly, spoke well, and handled his body better. He ran vigorously but awkwardly.

We have seen a number of very young children—seriously developmentally retarded and psychologically ill—whose mothers were seriously depressed during the first year after their birth.

Prevention and intervention during the first year of life may be one of the most important tasks of the mental health centers' children's programs. Paraprofessionals can be trained for routine visits to all new mothers. Their involvement with mothers leads to referral for help of those with persistent depression—an important preventive measure. Paraprofessionals can also ensure that new parents attend early evening classes with their babies. Each class focuses on developmental processes and the parents' facilitating roles in the child's development. Various age-appropriate stimulation techniques are demonstrated with the babies brought to the classes. The infants' obvious enjoyment at being sung to, talked with, and handled physically to encourage grasping, reaching, crawling, etc. stimulates parents to imitate the demonstrations at home.[29,36-39]

The child development classes provide opportunities for a child development specialist to see many babies and to refer some for more thorough developmental, neurophysiological examination. This permits early identification of minimally brain-damaged infants. Help and counseling for parents may prevent psychotic reactions. Without help, the parents' coping abilities are so severely tried that the parents also become disturbed.

In several centers the high-risk infants—those born blind, deaf, with cerebral palsy or cleft palate—are similarly worked with so parents can carry on home programs. These efforts are designed to fully utilize all the babies' potentials in intact areas. Hopeful and purposeful parent-child interaction reduces the emotional disturbances which result from the parents' helpless and hopeless feelings. These feelings are often manifested in desperate pushing of the child toward unrealizable normal functioning with resulting emotional disturbance and more retarded functioning.[40-42]

Both failure to thrive in the first year of life (resulting from parental emotional disturbance and anger at having a demanding infant, leading to depression and failure to feed the infant) and failure to grow (due to poverty and malnourishment following low birth weight) can be detected by public health nurses who make routine postpartum visits. Thus the community mental health center can lend its expertise in consultation and in-service training to the public health nurse or home-community worker so that close observation may permit helping services to be introduced and prevent nutritional deprivation of the infant and abuse of the child. [12,30,43,44]

In a few communities family planning has been made available through the health and mental health centers working together. They also collaborate to persuade pregnant women to attend the health center for prenatal checkups and to join jointly sponsored groups to discuss pregnancy and childbirth. These groups help parents who are depressed and have no one to turn to for help with such feelings. Several pilot projects demonstrate that depressed mothers are eager for help. The group reduces depression. After the baby's birth the group meetings can be supplemented with home visits to help these mothers learn techniques of handling the baby which permit mother and child to develop a good relationship.

The distribution of maternal depression across all socioeconomic classes makes such efforts by mental health centers in collaboration with health services important preventive measures.

Preschool Child Preventive Mental Health or Early Crisis Intervention

The classes in child development and the home visits by public health nurses, child development specialists, and paraprofessionals are all important in helping parents and children develop good relationships and facilitating the nurturance required by the infant for growth of competence, curiosity, and a capacity for learning. [12,15]

Such efforts have helped identify early problems, both physical and psychological, so that early intervention can occur. As the child becomes ambulatory, learns to speak, and becomes more independent, mothers who have enjoyed their relationship with a responsive infant may find the negativistic 2-year-old difficult to handle at home. Much child abuse occurs at this age, and many mothers begin to react to the walking, talking 2-year-old as a little adult. It therefore becomes important that parents learn to stay involved with their preschool children and have some relief from them. [45,46]

One of the most effective preventive programs described is a toddlers' preschool which provides group experiences for the child and an opportunity for parents to learn by participating as teachers' helpers in the preschool. A toy library and a good library of preschool books are helpful to the child's learning and maintain parents' involvement with their child. As part of a total program these efforts help parents to understand the problems and developmental issues during the 2- to 3-year period. [47,48,48a]

These preschool efforts at age 2 years help mothers left alone at home with their children to find a community of interests with other mothers through day-care centers with baby-sitting services. They also make the transition to nursery school an easier one for those children and mothers who are continuing participants. They begin a relationship to the child's learning in school with parents' participation in school as helpers in the classroom and concerned, informed participants in their child's learning through at least elementary school.[49]

Parents thus involved in their children's learning continue to provide stimulation to their children. Further, their concern with their child's learning has been shown by widely replicated research to be the single most important factor in their child's doing well in school and continuing to learn easily and well.[29]

The mental health implications are great. Children who learn and who feel competent tend to be mentally healthy. It is not accidental that more than 70 percent of children referred to child guidance or psychiatric clinics are referred for learning and behavior problems in school. Parents also feel better about themselves as parents and have fewer conflicts with their children as they understand and facilitate their offsprings' learning and total development.

Parents who are developmentally oriented can help teachers accept the need for more motor activity and motor learning opportunities for children—especially boys—who are large muscled or have a high activity rate.

In several programs the most effective teachers' aides have been parents who continued to be involved in their children's learning at home and in school and discovered their talents in teaching and working with children.

Developmental Evaluation in Preschool

The regular pediatric evaluations, or well-child care provided by nurse practitioners, as well as observations made by the home visitors, usually paraprofessionals, must be geared to assessing with parents the child's physical, cognitive, and social-emotional development. During the preschool period it becomes possible for educators to evaluate a large sample of children and to pick up developmental deviations which point to mild mental retardation or to neurophysiological dysfunction manifested in clumsiness, learning problems, problems in hand-eye coordination, or great emotional lability which may be predictive of neurophysiological deficits and which require precise diagnosis. Beginning remediation is possible with stimulant medication and through special attention and help to parents in starting special programs of interaction with their child to enhance existing ego functions and to improve areas where deficits in the child's physiological function exist.[22,47,48,48a]

Such early identification treatment and help to families which is sustained through the center can prevent the severe emotional disturbances common to these handicapped youngsters and their adverse effects on the entire family.

CASE EXAMPLE

Danny, at age 2 years, 6 months, was known to be slow in learning and was only now beginning to say a few words. His gait was clumsy and he seemed unable to use his hands to manipulate toys and blocks. He dropped most objects. Only his preschool teacher's repeated concern led his parents to take him to the pediatric clinic, where the history of a prolonged and difficult birth with anoxia, coupled with the slow development and recent increase in temper tantrums led to developmental testing and a neurological examination. He tested out developmentally as 1 year retarded. His motor clumsiness and incoordination confirmed the diagnosis of neurophysiological handicap. Specific stimulant medication, exercises, and a behavior modification program were instituted to help him learn and to help his parents help him control his temper.

A year later his retardation was still evident, but he was more sociable, learned with greater eagerness, and handled his body and hands more skillfully. Most notably his parents felt easier about him and did not need to give in to his complaining cries or spend so much time placating him, to the anger of their other children. These children had suffered relative neglect and had previously tried to hurt Danny when no one was looking. Now they worked with Danny, assured that their parents had time for them. Thus not only was Danny helped, but the parents were slowly educated about how he would develop. They saw his needs in the perspective of the family's needs. The mental health of Danny, parents, and siblings was greatly enhanced by the early diagnosis, intervention, and comprehensive attention to the family by the health–mental health team.

Education of Professionals and Paraprofessionals in Child Development

Most health and mental health professionals are poorly trained in the integration of physical development as known to the pediatrician, cognitive development as studied by some child psychologists, and affective social development reflected in developmental ego psychology as studied by child psychiatrists. A synthesis of developmental knowledge, a careful study of normative crisis periods during development, and understanding of the concepts of critical periods during which time certain physical and social development optimally occurs are necessary. [14,34,36a,47,50-52]

Developmental behavior originates during critical periods. If delayed by physical illness or psychological trauma, it is unlikely to develop fully. For example, if attachment behavior in the first 6 months of life, as described by Bowlby, is interfered with, affective and social development are unlikely to proceed without major difficulties throughout life. Basic trust of other human beings may never be solidly acquired. [34,53,53a]

The synthesis of developmental knowledge can be taught to all professionals for their daily use in understanding and working with children and families, and operationally, development can be taught to paraprofessionals. They can help assess physical, affective, social, and cognitive development through simplified testing and observations which can alert pediatricians, nurse practitioners, and preschool and primary-grade teachers to carry out more thorough evaluations leading to more expert diagnosis and early interventions. [36]

Crisis Intervention and Comprehensive Care: A Community Mental Health Center Concern

In working with the health care of preschool children and their families it is important that comprehensive family care become the goal. This means that the health care professional and mental health professional must collaborate to understand any serious or chronic illness in any family member as affecting family equilibrium with a potentially decompensating effect on other family members.[14,35,39]

CASE EXAMPLE

In one family the mother was discovered to have severe diabetes and needed to be hospitalized. To deal with this family crisis, the efforts of the team to alert preschool and other teachers of the children and to work with the father in terms of the demands and stress it would place on him and the children paid off. The teachers were able to talk with the children about their anxieties about the mother. The father was counseled, and the entire family met with the mother when she came home to help maintain her medication and diet. An exacerbation of the mother's illness was first picked up by the elementary-school teacher when one child, who began to do poor schoolwork, was gently questioned about it. She said her mother seemed sick again and stayed in bed a lot but didn't want to see the doctor and be hospitalized. A home visit by the public health nurse resulted in the mother's coming to the clinic, undergoing tests, and having her medication altered.

Everyone on the health–mental health–education–welfare team plays a vital part in the crisis intervention and the comprehensive care which enable sick family members to get better care and other family members to function better under stress. In this family both parents reported that the family's open discussions with mental health professionals about the effect of the mother's illness on the family began a pattern of their talking together about other family matters. To the parents' amazement, their children's comments were often wise, and their observations of how family members behaved were astute without being derogatory.

The School as a Mental Health Resource

The school is the first setting where all children are available for potential early diagnosis and remediation by education and health and mental health professionals. It sustains an influence over many children during their formative years and provides many unutilized opportunities to serve children and their families. Ideally the educational task is to deal with the whole child, his emotional as well as intellectual development. In reality emotional development is more and more of a problem to schools. Emotional development is often not seen as an issue at all.[41a]

Since the ratio of children to teachers is about 26:1, and that of children to mental health personnel 3660:1 for psychiatrists and 1050:1 for social workers, the mental health clinics see 1 out of 14 disturbed children; the schools see them all.[7,27,46,54]

Thus a mental health center that works closely with schools can, through mental health consultation and through early diagnostic services and use of paraprofessionals, have an enormous impact on child health and mental health problems. The mental health center as a collaborative institution can begin to educate colleagues in school about the normal crises of development (mother-child separations on school entry, entry into junior high and puberty crises) with great benefit to child and teacher.

It is clear that problem children in school find the school itself a problem for them. It is therefore important that a mental health center utilize the behavioral knowledge and skills of its staff to enhance the service delivery capacity of the schools.

Only about 6 percent of all mental health centers render consultation and education services to schools. Most of these existing services are for diagnosis and evaluation of severe behavioral disorders and therapeutic work with disturbed children. The consultation and education services of a collaborative type in which both school and mental health center personnel try together to work with the same children are rare.[42] Such collaboration needs to be a more common objective of both systems for mutual education and services to children.[8,55-59]

Learning and Acquiring Skills: A Mental Health Activity

The acquisition of basic skills and knowledge which makes employment likely and informed citizen involvement possible are prerequisite to mental health. Currently much of education is not meaningful. Material is not taught in a way to help children increase their interest in knowing and learning and to stimulate their curiosity and investigativeness.

In a few communities the educational system is engaged with the community in assessing the effectiveness of what it does and how it does it.[10] It is increasingly clear that the primary goal of education should be to help children learn skills and concepts basic to problem solving. Problem-solving methods are the single most helpful technique that can be learned in school, the most important capacity to be nurtured.

EXAMPLES

In one ghetto community a few parents, after much difficulty, succeeded in becoming involved in the elementary-school classrooms to ensure that their children, who usually dropped out or were kicked out in the third or fourth grade, really began to learn rather than sit in the classroom. They regularly worked in their youngsters' classrooms, helped reduce disruptive behavior, and worked to aid nonlearning students begin to acquire the rudiments of reading and arithmetic. These fairly sophisticated parents were angered because the teaching methods were so dull and asked some cadet teachers from the local teachers' college if learning to read and to do arithmetic could not be made more interesting and challenging. Two of the student-teachers had been working on a "project method" of teaching and learning about which they were excited. They presented their ideas to the parents and the principal in a meeting. The parents wanted the method tried. The principal was interested but cautious because he felt his teachers might feel threatened. Two young third- and fourth-grade teachers were willing to learn, and with the help of the cadet teachers, to work out the plans. The new teaching method was introduced.

As described in several publications,[60] youngsters who became interested in the third and fourth grade in a project like history of baseball were divided into small groups to investigate certain aspects of their chosen project. One small group focused on black baseball players, another on the Baseball Hall of Fame, another on the greatest hitters in baseball. The small groups slowly had to learn to work together, decide how to get the information and put it together using their teachers as resource persons. They were helped to write letters, to read books, to learn how to compute batting averages and to compile reports into a volume on the history of baseball. The local black newspaper sportswriter became a resource person for one group and showed them how to get information on Satchel Page, the famous black pitcher. The degree of learning in reading and math was astounding.

When parents and interested teachers in the local junior high school insisted that they also use project learning, they found it equally stimulating to students. In addition to learning to work together in groups these students learned how democracy works in practice in the classroom. Teachers helped them through the projects they chose on urban renewal, juvenile delinquency, etc. They learned to do research, gather data, and present their findings from which they drew conclusions. In the classroom many decisions were made in the same way, with teachers acting as resource persons.

The students ran into trouble when their data on urban renewal revealed that these efforts did not help people in the ghetto, but only made things worse. Their excellent presentations to a parent group annoyed the city urban renewal office, which reacted to the excellent research with anger and questioned this learning method's relevancy for junior-high-school students. With parent help other classes began project research, only to run into opposition from teachers who were threatened rather than challenged by the eagerness of students to learn to gather data and assess and draw conclusions through class discussions.

In another school district teachers were concerned with how children could be helped in adolescence to understand their own mixed feelings, their confusion about sex, human relations, and parenthood. They sought to use a nearby day-care center as a way to teach human development which would lead to talking about human feelings, human physiology, and anatomy as part of development. This project led students to explore and collect information about reproductive physiology and sexual customs in other societies also as part of human development. They spent 4 hours a week working with 2- to 5-year-old children. This led to easier interaction with the children and between the boys and girls involved in project learning in each of the areas mentioned. These youngsters in a poor, ethnically mixed neighborhood became the best informed junior-high-school students about development, human physiology and reproduction, and how to work with small children. In their cooperative efforts they acquired easy working relationships with each other. Respect for each other among the boys and girls became clear and they also revealed empathy for each others' feelings as they found they could talk more openly about feelings and experiences in the classroom.

These youngsters also learned the problem-solving methods of gathering information, assessing information for validity, and then, through discussion, reaching reasonable conclusions.

In these schools mental health problems as measured by behavior problems, failure in school, dropping out, or expulsion, were greatly reduced.

How mental health centers lend their personnel to stimulate and help in such efforts is a current concern of those interested in prevention of failure in school. There is little question that failure in school leads to leaving school, becoming part of a street culture, and inevitably becoming involved in delinquent acts and drugs. The data on the students just described are not yet available, but from other work it is clear that young people with a sense of self-competence and a good self-image tend to be less involved in drugs and crime and to have clearer goals for themselves. Also, as parents stay interested in their children's learning they help them succeed in school and plan for meaningful work and education.[7,60a]

The role of education in helping students learn the methods of solving problems can lead to more active, involved, and informed citizen participation. This is the antithesis of the helpless-hopelessness common to many depressed, powerless-feeling adults.

The Role of Work in Prevention of Mental Illness

It is clear from the studies of the Leightons and others that jobs and meaningful work are essential to good mental health. For young adults to have a meaningful education, part of their learning must be work-oriented. They need to learn to do effectively a job that fits their interests and temperament. The health and mental health care and educational systems can provide opportunities for learning jobs that are important to the community and the individual.[32,61]

The prevention orientation of a mental health center includes its consultation and educational function to other agencies: schools, welfare, industry, and city-county agencies. Helping other agencies become aware of the mental health implications of work will also help them explore ways of finding meaningful employment for the adolescents and young adults in the community.[37,41,55,56,62,63]

Special Education and the Mental Health Center

Too often mental health centers are so closely tied to an old therapeutic model that they fail to recognize the relevance of educational efforts for developmentally disabled (neurologically and physically impaired) and the emotionally disturbed students in their community.

Special schools like Project Re-Ed for moderately disturbed children or the League School for psychotic children in New York, have great therapeutic impact through the educational process. The schools developed in various Kennedy centers for the retarded have pointed the way to keeping developmentally disabled children meaningfully in the home with less emotional disturbance for themselves and their families.

Mental Health Consultation: An Intervention and Prevention Tool

All mental health centers are enjoined to provide mental health consultation services and education to agencies in their community. Few have either the trained personnel or the time and commitment to siphon personnel away from direct services and use them for mental health consultation.

It is currently clear that mental health consultation to special education classes permits teachers to work more effectively with deviant children they would otherwise get rid of. Similarly, schools in general, juvenile courts, welfare services, and protective services require consultation to understand how their particular efforts can more effectively alter the behavior of children and youth they would ordinarily abandon.

One of the most important aspects of consultation is that it helps other professionals do their jobs better by enabling them to understand the problems and to find idiosyncratic ways of helping a disturbed and disturbing child to function better.[37,41,55,56,63,63a,63b] Group consultation to teachers, probation officers, and welfare workers enhances the capacities of these fellow professionals to work easily and effectively with a wide spectrum of clients.

EXAMPLE

In one ghetto junior high school, group consultation with the teachers disclosed their sense of impotence in dealing with the nonlearning, disruptive student. One teacher volunteered to describe a student and try to work with him according to the plan we worked out. In the process of gathering the data about this boy, we came to understand the impact on a family of moving to the West from the Deep South. We came to recognize how the failure to help this bright boy to learn occurred from kindergarten on because his size and belligerence caused teachers to avoid him. Now in the eighth grade, school still meant something to him because he kept coming to class although he still had learned little. From the data obtained in her only contact (made at our request) with the mother, who otherwise avoided school because her son was in constant trouble, the teacher learned that he was a good mechanic and helped older boys in the neighborhood work on their cars. The teacher was then encouraged by the group to use a third-grade reader on auto repairs to begin to teach him to read. The 15 minutes she spent with him morning and afternoon were the first quiet periods he had spent in that classroom. He slowly learned to read because of his interest in cars. His math was first centered on measuring bearings and the tolerances in gears on which the classroom teacher had to gather information from the shop teacher. She gradually helped him to figure out gear ratios until he became fairly proficient in math. During the semester we followed this youngster there were many ups and downs, but many of the teachers in the group could see the general trend toward improvement and began to collect data on the difficult students in their classes and to discuss the implications of these findings for different ways of reaching their students through more attuned and individualized teaching.

THE MENTAL HEALTH SERVICES
SPECTRUM FOR CHILDREN

Crisis Intervention

One of the most meaningful services a center can provide is crisis intervention. A crisis in a family is an opportunity for utilizing the energies mobilized in each individual and in the family to resolve some family problems. If the crisis goes untreated, consolidation occurs, with a general decrease in the family's ability to function. Instead of learning how to handle stress as a family, the members suffer its disorganizing effect and are less resistant to new stress.[68]

The activity required of the helpers often serves to mobilize the individuals who have felt helpless. Thus in a crisis of severe illness in a child, the example of the mental health professional in openly discussing the illness and its prognosis and answering questions readily serves as a model for family interaction. In addition, a task-oriented approach which requires certain behavior on the part of family members to reduce the crisis promotes action rather than helplessness. In the case of the severely ill child, parents can be helped to divide time spent with the sick child to allow more time with the other children at home so they don't feel abandoned and forced to act out to gain parents' attention. The other siblings are encouraged to help parents by performing those chores realistic to their capabilities. Increased family communication through regular meetings during the illness and death of a child permits open expression of feelings and open mourning. Appropriate weeping is encouraged rather than repression of sorrow. When such behavior is enhanced by openly expressed concerns of the alerted teacher to the children, greater openness occurs in the family. The increased energy and openness of feeling thus brought about also permit the dying child to feel supported by each parent, who can nurture him more freely. Such a family may find itself better able to feel openly and to communicate together after such a crisis event.[35,39,51,64-67]

Therapeutic Schools and Day-Care Centers

We have already mentioned models of therapeutic schools for children. Often needed are therapeutic nursery schools and elementary schools geared to providing a therapeutic milieu around learning. Such a milieu takes cognizance of the distractibility of disturbed children and their need to develop relationships with adults and other children. A large adult/child ratio is necessary to permit a wide variety of learning activities facilitated by the relationships with well-trained adults. Learning activities are aimed at enhancing body image through dance and athletics, socialization through cooperative building projects, capacity to increase normal skills through occupational therapy projects with clay, paint, nails, and wood leading to skilled activities like model building. Every activity is aimed at enhancing the child's sense of self-worth and increasing his competence in learning and relationships.[67a]

Each school setting must include parents who, by observing trained adults working with their child and other children, learn to work more effectively with their child at home.[68]

Most therapeutic day-care centers and schools also provide individual diagnostic and therapeutic services to children.

Regular day-care centers can have special classes designed to provide therapeutic impact on less disturbed children who need help either before or after school. These classes are especially designed to give personalized attention to children with learning problems and to use small activity groups to enhance socialization and develop observational skills, attention span, and manual skills.

Outpatient Services

Local outpatient services to provide individual and group therapy for children and parents are prerequisite to effective treatment programs.

Many children's programs have found that latency-age children and adolescents do very well in group therapy designed to meet the activity level and interests of the child population.

Parent-education groups for all the children's services are important. Parents who meet together to understand their children's problems feel less alone, and they feel better understood by other parents than by professionals. Educational efforts to help parents learn to manage their children are often useful. Those parents who require individual aid because of their degree of disturbance also learn and contribute a great deal in the group setting, thus enhancing their self-worth.[68]

Day Hospital Care

Experience has shown that separation of child and parents for long periods of time is disruptive to the parent-child relationship and detrimental to the child's improvement. For disturbed children who require medication and a very structured program to integrate them during a psychotic episode, a day hospital is relatively inexpensive and promotes improvement leading to easy transfer to a therapeutic day-care center.

Parents of such youngsters do well in a therapeutic day-care center parent-education group. Many of these parents can be encouraged to work in the day hospital so they become familiar with its activities, its structure, and the attitudes of staff which promote their child's greater integration. We have used an electronic bug-in-the-ear technique to give instructions to parents working with their own and other children on well-defined and structured tasks. This technique helps them over moments of helplessness, withdrawal, or anger which create distance between parent and child. Parents' work with their child is important to the child's improvement.

Inpatient Care

A few children with severe psychoses require 24-hour care. Inpatient care is best used on a temporary basis to help drugs take hold and to permit experienced personnel to help the child to settle down. Most children can be transferred to day hospital or therapeutic day care in a few days to a few weeks. However, the lack of such facilities makes it difficult to treat the few such children in a community. Usually treatment must be given at a state hospital or on an adult ward, both frightening and disorganizing experiences for a sick child.[68]

Group Homes and Foster Homes

Sometimes the home situation is too unstable, or parental desertion, death of a parent, or a new marriage makes the home unsuitable for the child temporarily or permanently. These youngsters need the experience of a group home on a temporary basis when there is some likelihood of the family reconstituting after a period of crisis.

The foster home where a number of disturbed children are cared for by experienced foster parents, is a viable alternative to the real home only when the foster parents have been carefully selected and when they agree to work regularly with the consultants of the center.

Both group homes and foster homes, to be effective, must have a spectrum of services regularly provided. The most important service is regular follow-up of each child with the surrogate parents so that problems can be anticipated and worked through. The consultation model of helping the surrogate parents as coprofessionals to do their job better through enhanced understanding and closely followed interventions creates truly professional and effective surrogate parents. Other services like home teaching and occupational-recreational services are important to the improvement of many seriously disturbed children.

A Team Approach to Services

The success of service programs depends upon their integration so that teams of therapists and teachers follow children from school and home into any treatment service and out.

A team which works with one child and forms a close and effective collaborative relationship over time is the most economical way of utilizing professional personnel. The team of mental health professional and teacher can help other personnel in temporary relationships with a child to understand him developmentally. It can identify and help others understand the child's ego capacities and those areas of ego functioning which are temporarily lost. The focus can then be on helping the child to regain functions and to acquire new ones.

A schoolteacher who is part of a mental health team finds it easier to work with a disturbed child in the regular classroom as part of the effort to return the child to normal functioning.

Function of Supportive Networks

In a few centers the community networks of Y's, recreational, religious, and other supports can be utilized to help provide experiences important to the child's more normal functioning.

In one community retired elderly men and women were enlisted to work with youngsters in neighborhood facilities on individual projects to promote their curiosity, attention, and learning. Several of these elderly persons not only became skillful in helping disturbed children by their devoted individual care but also alerted the center when the child got worse, and in a number of instances picked up disturbances in children not yet identified by the school or health care agency.

The coordination of services on behalf of a child and family may require a special advocate from the health–mental health agency who makes sure that the prescribed services get to the child and that paperwork and other bureaucratic obstacles do not delay or prevent delivery of services.[69]

EVALUATION

Methods of evaluating the effectiveness of services are developing. In essence these methods all depend on written assessment of the problems and their severity, a developmental and functional diagnosis of areas of nonfunctioning, a description of the treatment program to be carried out, and a prediction of the outcome for each child patient and family. Outcome must be described in terms of how the child and family will be able to function on discharge and, with the treatment program prescribed, how long it should take. Such information allows objective evaluation, forces examination of outcome, and enables learning from prediction.

Prevention programs are more difficult to evaluate. However, when one works with depressed mothers or unstimulated children, the effect of the interventions can be recorded and compared with already documented experiences with infants and mothers who have not been helped.[70-72] Hopefully, the thrust in most mental health centers will be more toward prevention and early intervention despite the constant pressure for treatment services.

SUMMARY

Most mental health services attend primarily to the most vocal and disturbing members of their catchment areas: the adult mentally ill. In a few mental health centers with a commitment to children, new early intervention and prevention services have been successfully initiated. Such early prevention and intervention services to children and their families are highly important. Poverty, malnutrition, and maternal depression account for much mental illness in the first few years of life. Methods of prevention and early intervention have been worked out and are available.

Mental health centers must focus on these methods and must now look carefully at the increasing numbers of disturbed and nonlearning, delinquent and drug-taking children in all socioeconomic classes. These children are their potential adult patients. Parent involvement with children's early learning and stimulation, and the use of paraprofessionals as case finders and helpers in interventions are ways of preventing health and mental health problems.

The school as a source of collaboration between education, health, and mental health is crucial for the welfare of all children.

REFERENCES

1. Deutscher I: The social causes of social problems: From suicide to delinquency. In Mizruchi HE (ed): The Substance of Sociology. New York, Appleton, 1967

1a. Special section: Inner city mental health services. Am J Psychiatry 126:1430–1480, 1970

1b. Rexford EN: Children, child psychiatry, and our brave new world. Arch Gen Psychiatry 20:25–37, 1969

2. Kellam SG, Schiff SK: An urban community mental health center. In Duhl L, Leopold R (eds): Mental Health and Urban Social Policy: A Casebook of Community

Actions. San Francisco, Jossey-Bass, 1968

3. Kellam SG, Schiff, SK: The Woodlawn Mental Health Center: A community mental health center model. Soc Service Rev 40:255–263, 1966

4. Minuchin S, Montalvo B: Techniques for working with disorganized low socioeconomic families. Am J Orthopsychiatry 37:880–887, 1967

5. Rafferty FT: The community is becoming. Am J Orthopsychiatry 36:102–110, 1966

6. Minuchin S: The paraprofessional and the use of confrontation in the mental health field. Am J Orthopsychiatry 39:722–729, 1969

7. US Department of Health, Education, and Welfare: Mental Health and Learning: When Community Mental Health Centers and School Systems Collaborate. DHEW Publication No (HSM) 72-9146. Washington, DC, GPO, 1972

8. US Department of Health, Education, and Welfare: Mental Health Consultation to Programs for Children: A Review of Data Collected from Selected U.S. Sites. Public Health Service Publication No 2066. Washington, DC, GPO, 1970

9. Bower EM: Early Identification of Emotionally Handicapped Children in School. Springfield Ill, Thomas, 1960

10. Bower EM: The modification, mediation and utilization of stress during the school years. Am J Orthopsychiatry 34:667–674, 1964

11. Berlin IN: Resistance to change in mental health professionals. Am J Orthopsychiatry 39:109–115, 1969

12. Braun S: The well baby clinic: Its prospects for building ego strength. Am J Public Health 55:1889–1898, 1965

13. Call J D: Prevention of autism in a young infant in a well-child conference. J Am Acad Child Psychiatry 2:451–459, 1963

14. Caplan G: The role of pediatrics in community mental health. In Bellak L (ed): Handbook of Community Psychiatry and Community Mental Health. New York, Grune & Stratton, 1964

15. Cary AC, Reveal M T: Prevention and detection of emotional disturbances in preschool children. Am J Orthopsychiatry 37:719–724, 1967

16. Klebanoff L B, Bindman AJ: The organization and development of a community mental health program for children: A case study. Am J Orthopsychiatry 32:119–132, 1962

17. Malone CA: Children. In Grunebaum H (ed): The Practice of Community Mental Health. Boston, Little Brown, 1970

17a. Westman JC, Rice DL, Bermann E: Nursery school behavior and later school adjustment. Am J Orthopsychiatry 37:725–731, 1967

18. Cravioto J, Delicarie ER, Birch HG: Nutrition, growth, and neuro-integrative development: An experimental and ecologic study. Pediatrics 38(2) suppl, 1966

19. Scrimshaw NS: Infant malnutrition and adult learning. Saturday Rev Lit 51:64–67, 1968

20. Scrimshaw NS, Guzman MA, Gordon J E: Nutrition and infection field study in Guatemalan villages. Arch Environ Health 14:657–662, 1967

21. Stoch MB: Undernutrition during infancy and subsequent brain growth and intellectual development. In Scrimshaw N S, Gordon JE (eds): Malnutrition: Learning and Behavior. Cambridge, Mass, MIT Press, 1968

22. Birch HG: The problem of "brain damage" in children. In Birch HG (ed): Brain Damage in Children: The Biological and Social Aspects. Baltimore, Williams & Wilkins, 1964.

23. Cassel J: Social class and mental disorders: An analysis of the limitations and potentialities of current epidemiological approaches. In Miller KS, Grigg CM (eds): Mental Health and the Lower Class. Tallahassee, Florida State University Press, 1966

24. Pasamanick B, Knobloch H, Lillienfeld AM: and reproductive casualty. Am J Orthopsychiatry 30:298, 1960

25. Pasamanick B, Knobloch H, Lillienfeld AM: Socioeconomic status and some precursors of neuropsychiatric disorders. Am J Orthopsychiatry 26:594–601, 1956

26. Srole L, Langer TS, Michael ST, Opler MK, Rennie, TA: Mental Health in the Metropolis: The Midtown Manhattan Study, vol I. New York, McGraw-Hill, 1962

27. Werner EE, Bierman J, French FE: Children of Kauai. Honolulu, University of Hawaii Press, 1971

28. Wiener G, Rider RV, Oppel WC, Fisch-

er LK, Harper PA: Correlates of low birth weight: Psychological status at six to seven years of age. Pediatrics 35:434–444, 1965

29. Crow M: Preventive intervention through parent group education. Soc Casework 67:161–165, 1967

30. Leonard MF, Rhymes JP, Solnit AJ: Failure to thrive in infants. Am J Dis Child 111:600–612, 1966

31. Schwartz LH, Snider J, Schwartz JE: Psychiatric case report of nutritional battering with implications for community agencies. Community Ment Health J 3:163–169, 1967

32. Leighton D, Harding JS, Macklin DB, Macmillan AM, Leighton AH: The Character of Danger. New York, Basic Books, 1963

33. Ainsworth MD: The effects of maternal deprivation: A review of findings and controversy in the context of research strategy. WHO Public Health Pap 4:97–165, 1962

34. Bowlby J: Attachment and Loss, vol 1: Attachment. New York, Basic Books, 1969

35. Cadden V: Crisis in the family. In Caplan G (ed): Principles of Preventive Psychiatry. New York, Basic Books, 1964

36. Bayley N, Schaefer ES: Maternal behavior, child behavior, and their intercorrelations from infancy through adolescence. Monogr Soc Res Child Dev 28(3), 1963

36a. Reiff R, Riessman F: The indigenous nonprofessional: A strategy of change in community action and community mental health programs. Community Ment Health J (Monograph 1), 1965

37. Berlin IN: Prevention of mental and emotional disorders in childhood. In Wolman B B (ed): Manual of Child Psychopathology. New York, McGraw-Hill, 1972

38. Brim OG Jr: Education for Child Rearing. New York, Russell Sage Foundation, 1959

39. Caplan G: Patterns of parental response to the crisis of premature birth. Psychiatry 23:365–374, 1960

40. Ambrosino S: A project in group education with parents of retarded children. In Casework Papers. New York, Family Service Association of America, 1960

41. Berlin IN: Consultation and special education. In Philips I (ed): Prevention and Treatment of Mental Retardation. New York,, Basic Books, 1966

42. Philips I (ed): Prevention and Treatment of Mental Retardation. New York, Basic Books, 1966

43. Bullard DM Jr, Glaser HH, Heagarty MC, Pivchik E: Failure to thrive in the "neglected" child. Am J Orthopsychiatry 37:680–690, 1967

44. Green M, Solnit A: Reactions to the threatened loss of a child: A vulnerable child syndrome. Pediatrics 34:58, 1964

45. Kiesler F: More than psychiatry: A rural program. In Shore MF, Mannino FV (eds): Mental Health and the Community: Problems, Programs, and Strategies. New York, Behavioral Publications, 1969

46. Zax M, Cowen EL: Early identification and prevention of emotional disturbance in a public school. In Cowen EL, Gardner EA, Zax M (eds): Emergent Approaches to Mental Health Problems. New York, Appleton, 1967

47. Hess RD, Shipman VC: Early experience and the socialization of cognitive modes in children. Child Res 36:869–886, 1965

48. Kagan J, Moss HA, Sigel IE: Psychological significance of styles of conceptualization. Monogr Soc Res Child Dev 28(2):73–112, 1963

48a. Weiss G, Mind K, Werry JS, Douglas V, Nemeth E: Studies on the hyperactive child: Five year follow-up. Arch Gen Psychiatry, 24:409–414, May 1971

49. White RW: Motivation reconsidered: The concept of competence. Psychol Rev 66(5):297–333, 1959

50. Lewis WW: Project Re-Ed: Educational intervention in discordant child rearing systems. In Cowen EL, Gardner EA, Zax M (eds): Emergent Approaches to Mental Health Problems. New York, Appleton, 1967

51. Parad HJ: The use of time-limited crisis intervention in community mental health programming. Soc Service Rev 40:275–282, 1966

52. Prugh DG, Staub EM, Sands HH, Kirschbaum RM, Lenihan EA: A study of the emotional reactions of children and families to hospitalization and illness. Am J Orthopsychiatry 23:70–106, 1953

53. Scott JP: Critical periods in behavioral development. Science 138:949–955, 1962

53a. Korner AF, Grobstein R: Visual alertness as related to soothing in neonates: Implications for maternal stimulation and early deprivation. Child Dev 37:867–876, 1966

54. Whittington HG: Institutional lodgement of the comprehensive community mental health center. Am J Public Health 59:451–458, 1969

55. Berlin IN: Learning mental health consultation: History and problems. Ment Hyg 48:257–266, 1964

56. Berlin IN: Mental health consultation for school social workers: A conceptual model. Community Ment Health J 5:280–288, 1969

57. Berlin IN: Preventive aspects of mental health consultation to schools. Ment Hyg 51:34–40, 1967

58. Iscoe I, Pierce-Jones J, Friedman ST, McGehearty L: Some strategies in mental health consultation: A brief description of a project and some preliminary results. In Cowen EL, Gardner EA, Zax M (eds): Emergent Approaches to Mental Health Problems. New York, Appleton, 1967

59. Sheldon A: On consulting to new, changing, or innovative organizations. Community Ment Health J 7:62–71, 1971

60. Berlin IN: The school's role in a participatory democracy. Am J. Orthopsychiatry 42:499–507, 1972

60a. Ojemann RH: Investigations on the effects of teaching an understanding and appreciation of behavior dynamics. In Caplan G (ed): Prevention of Mental Disorders in Children. New York, Basic Books, 1961

61. Silber E, Coelho G, Murphey E, Hamburg D, Pearlin L, Rosenberg M: Competent adolescents coping with college decisions. Arch Gen Psychiatry 5:517–527, 1961

62. Bolman WM, Westmen JC: Prevention of mental disorder: An overview of current programs. Am J Psychiatry 123:1058–1068, 1967

63. Caplan G: Theory and Practice of Mental Health Consultation. New York, Basic

Books, 1970

63a. Coleman JR: Psychiatric consultation in casework agencies. Am J Orthopsychiatry 7:533–539, 1947

63b. Goldston SE: Mental Health education in a community mental health center. Am J Public Health 58:693–699, 1968

64. Berlin IN: Crisis intervention and short-term therapy. J Am Acad Child Psychiatry 9:595–606, 1970 Also in Barten HH, Barten SS (eds): Children and Their Parents in Brief Therapy. New York, Behavioral Publications, 1973

65. Mason EA: The hospitalized child: His emotional needs. N Engl J Med 272:406–414, 1965

66. Prouty RW, Prillaman D: Diagnostic teaching: A modest proposal. Elem School J 70(5):265–270, 1970

67. Rahe, RH, Meyer M, Smith M, Kjaer G, Holmes TH: Social stress and illness onset. J Psychom Res 8:34–44, 1964

67a. Bettelheim B: The Empty Fortress. New York, Free Press, 1967

68. Joint Commission on Mental Health of Children. Crisis in Child Mental Health. New York, Harper & Row, 1970

69. Schiff SK: Community accountability and mental health services. Ment Hyg 54:205–214, 1970

70. Hetznecker W, Forman MA: Community child psychiatry: Evolution and direction. Am J Orthopsychiatry 41:350–370, 1971

71. Harrison I, McDermott J, Schrager J, Showerman E: Social status and child psychiatric practice: The influence of the clinician's socioeconomic origin. Am J Psychiatry 127:652–658, 1970

72. Anthony EJ: Primary prevention with school children. In Barten HH, Bellak L (eds): Progress in Community Mental Health. New York, Grune & Stratton, 1972, Vol. 2, pp 131–138.

ADDITIONAL READINGS

Bellak L (ed): Handbook of Community Psychiatry and Community Mental Health. New York, Grune & Stratton, 1964

Bindman AJ, Klebanoff LB: Administrative

problems in establishing a community mental health clinic. Amer J Orthopsychiatry 30:696–711

Freed H, Miller L: Planning a community mental

health program: A case history. Community Ment Health J 7:107–117, 1971

Glascote R et al: The Community Mental Health Center: An Interim Appraisal. Washington, DC, American Psychiatric Association, 1969

Glueck S, Glueck E: Predicting Delinquency and Crime. Cambridge, Mass, Harvard University Press, 1959

Hobbs DB, Osman MP: From prison to the community. Crime Delinquency 13:317–322, 1967

Hume PB: General principles of community psychiatry. In Arieti S (ed): American Handbook of Psychiatry, vol 3. New York, Basic Books, 1966

Kvaraceus WC: Forecasting delinquency: A three-year-experiment. Except Child 27:429–435, 1961

Leininger M: Some anthropological issues related to community mental health programs in the United States. Community Ment Health J 7:24–28, 1971

Leopold R: Urban problems and the community mental health center: Multiple mandates, difficult choices. 1. Background and current status. Am J Orthopsychiatry 41:144–149, 1971

Niebuhr R. Without consensus there is no consent. The Center Magazine 4(4):2–9, 1971

Sarason S, Levine M, Goldenberg I, Cherlin DL, Bennett EM: Psychology in Community Settings. New York, Wiley, 1966

Skeels HM: Adult status of children with contrasting early life experiences: A follow-up study. Monogr Soc Res Child Dev 31(3, ser. no. 105), 1966

Stage TB, Keast T: A psychiatric service for plains Indians. Hosp Community Psychiatry 17:131–133, 1966

Herbert D. Kleber, M.D.

7

Drug Abuse

The use of certain psychoactive drugs for altering an individual's state of consciousness has occurred probably everywhere such drugs have been available. In some instances, drug use has remained limited to a few individuals who could then be labeled as deviant by the larger society. In other instances, it has become so widespread as to be a part of the cultural norm with no stigma attached to the users. In still other cases, and the United States is a good example of this category, there has been a combination of both of these. Certain drugs—alcohol, tobacco, and tranquilizers—achieved widespread use and were tolerated by society; others—heroin and lysergic acid diethylamide (LSD)—remained limited to a relatively few individuals or groups who were then labeled deviant; still another—marijuana—is widely used and yet its possession illegal. Use also varies in a culture from time to time in regard both to the types of drugs used and the part of the population using them.

We do not know whether the present extensive use of drugs in a nonprescription fashion is an epidemic that will subside as have some previous ones, whether it will stay the same, or whether it will greatly increase. We do not know whether current or future preventive and educational efforts will deter future users or whether efforts at legal control of drug availability will be more successful than they have been in the past or will simply shift the pattern of drug taking. We do not know whether certain kinds of drug use now illegal will receive social and legal sanction and increase. We can say with some certainty, however, that while the decision to use drugs is an individual one, the type and extent of drug usage are greatly influenced by community and national factors. We can also say that, regardless of the answers to the above questions, as long as drugs are used there will be some casualties of such use and it will remain necessary to provide humane and effective treatment for such individuals.

DEFINITIONS

In few medical fields are definitions as confusing as in the area of drug use, and in few areas do the definitions depend so much on the point of view of the speaker or writer. In order to keep such confusion to a minimum in this chapter, some key words and phrases are defined below, in terms of what they mean in this chapter and how others use them.

Drug. Technically this refers to any chemical taken to produce physical or psychological changes. In this chapter it refers specifically to a psychoactive substance used specifically for the purpose of altering one's psychological state. Although alcohol is clearly a drug by this definition, it is discussed in a separate chapter.

Drug use or usage. This refers to the purposeful taking of any psychoactive substance.

Illegal drug. This can be either a drug that cannot be purchased legally in this country except perhaps for research (heroin, LSD) or a drug that can be purchased legally with a doctor's prescription but has not been so obtained by the individual in question. Thus, if you borrow a few barbituates from your neighbor who got them from her doctor, you possess an illegal drug, your neighbor a legal one. In this chapter illegal drug refers to both possibilities: It means a drug which it is illegal for the particular individual to possess.

Drug abuse. This phrase is the most value-laden and confusing one in the whole area. To some it means the taking of a drug in any quantity or at any time not under medical auspices and/or for a medicinal purpose. The abuse lies in the intention of the user. Thus, an individual who takes a barbiturate under his doctor's orders to promote sleep is a drug user; if the same individual takes the same amount of barbiturate to promote not sleep but a "high" feeling, he is a drug abuser. Under this definition, any use of an illegal drug equals abuse. In this chapter a different definition is employed. Drug abuse means the nonprescription use of psychoactive chemicals by an individual to alter his psychological state in a situation in which the individual or society incurs some harm. Under this definition the occasional use of a drug, legal or not, in which no harm occurs is not drug abuse. The definition is perforce a medical one rather than a legal one; in the latter discipline, any use of an illegal drug could equal abuse.

Experimental, occasional, or recreational use. This is the sporadic or temporary use of drugs from which no harm is usually expected but which is viewed with concern by segments of society because it might lead to more regular use or because specific harm may occur, e.g., a psychotic reaction or an automobile accident.

Regular but moderate use.   This is continued use of certain drugs but in a pattern that does not have the pervasive aspects of the next category. The individual is regarded as being more at risk than the occasional user.

Dependence.   As defined by the World Health Organization this is "a state of psychic or physical dependence, or both, on a drug, arising in a person following administration of that drug on a periodic or continuous basis. The characteristics of such a state will vary with the agent involved."[1]

Many of the difficulties that hamper intelligent discussion of drug use stem from loose application of the above term, especially those having to do with patterns and frequency of use. In one of the commonest instances of this communication failure, one finds an adolescent defending the harmlessness of marijuana compared with alcohol, while the parent is defending the safety of alcohol and condemning marijuana as extremely dangerous. Close questioning often discloses that the adolescent is thinking of the occasional marijuana user versus the alcoholic, while the parent visualizes the moderate social drinker versus the chronically stoned social dropout using marijuana among many other drugs. In such situations rational discussion becomes next to impossible. Similarly, the adult who uses alcohol for enhancing recreation often cannot comprehend the teenager who uses marijuana at a party; the housewife who finds she can whip through her housekeeping chores when she takes a diet pill cannot understand her son who pops "speed" for the sense of energy and competence it gives him.

It is because of these and similar examples that some observers are beginning to talk about the drug-problem problem, to wonder whether much of the public concern—at times bordering on hysteria—is not misplaced and in fact exacerbates the problem. Unfortunately, like many other reactions to drug abuse, this one too appears exaggerated. Drugs can indeed be dangerous; too many Americans expose themselves to such dangers on an ill-informed basis; excessive use of legal drugs does not excuse excessive use of illegal drugs; and the numbers using illegal drugs increased markedly in the 1960s although a downturn appears now to be taking place. One cannot, therefore, ignore the problem and hope it will go away. While such benign neglect might reduce hysteria and excessive reactions that do more harm than good, it would probably also dry up the funding that for the first time since the 1920s has provided adequate treatment for the drug-scene casualties in this country. The emphasis in this chapter is on what an intelligent community mental health approach can and cannot do to remedy the problem without exacerbating it.

THEORIES ON THE CAUSE OF DRUG ABUSE

Not only is the cause of drug abuse not definitively known, but the various theories advanced are as often contradictory as they are complementary. In such a situation, the exact actions to be taken by community mental health programs are often unclear. To expand on this point it is useful to review briefly some suggested causes and the remedies that flow from acceptance of them as causative agents.

Availability.   The role of availability is often emphasized, since, of course, if drugs were not available, no one could abuse them. The high incidence of drug abuse among medical personnel and in inner-city areas is often cited as related to availability. If this is accepted as a primary cause, then the remedy is usually law enforcement or supply regulation. Supplies of illicit drugs entering the country or manufactured clandestinely must be cut off and diversion of legal drugs to the black market halted. Heroin maintenance is an offshoot of this theory, since it presumably would help dry up the black market. Availability can relate both to individual use (e.g., by physicians) and to epidemic use (e.g., the amphetamine epidemic in Japan after World War II).

Disease.   One popular model espoused by mental health professionals is that drug abuse is engendered by psychological problems in the host. Personality disturbances relating to dependence, handling of aggression, or sexual problems are cited, among others, as relevant factors.[2] If this is the case, then the remedy lies in psychological treatment for the individual abuser and a massive effort to improve psychological services for the community at large to decrease the incidence of those traits that lead to drug dependence. The epidemic quality of drug abuse at times is explained by asserting that there always exists in the population a high incidence of the relevant traits and that when availability increases, an epidemic ensues.

Socioeconomic factors.   The high incidence of drug abuse in ghetto areas— regardless of which minority group happens to be in the ghetto at the time—is often cited as showing that the major cause of drug abuse relates to poverty and the hopelessness that state often engenders.[3] The remedy then is to improve the socioeconomic status and outlook of the poor by means of improved housing, job opportunities, revision of the welfare structure. Epidemics are explained by insisting that the number of drug users has always been high and that the "epidemic" occurs not when numbers increase but when something happens to bring the problem to the attention of the affluent part of society, e.g., visible use in suburban communities or crime spilling out of the ghetto into affluent areas.

Social factors.   Attempts to find a single explanation for both inner-city and suburban drug use have popularized theories that blame drug abuse on the evils of American society. Such an explanation usually invokes problem areas such as economic inequality (or capitalism per se), racism, the Vietnam War, the military-industrial complex, excessive emphasis on materialism, and hypocrisy in government.[4] The remedies then involve remaking society by means of massive institutional change of either a revolutionary or an evolutionary variety.

Combinations.   Often two or more of the above factors are cited together, either as a general theory or as an attempt to explain a particular aspect of drug abuse. These combinations most often involve an external factor (e.g., availability, the mass media) with a factor relating to the individual himself (e.g., alienation, poverty).[3] The remedy suggested would then involve attacks on both sets of factors, although the emphasis usually is determined by the point of view of the speaker. Thus, when legal officials discuss addiction, they often pay at least lip service to the idea of factors affecting the individual, but the major stress is usually on availability, the crime associated with addiction, and the need for more resources in the criminal justice system. Similar results with different emphasis occur when mental health professionals or sociologists discuss drug abuse: Availability is mentioned but stress is on more money for housing, jobs, treatment.

A critical examination of all these points of view demonstrates that none has all the answers. Each sheds some light on one aspect of drug abuse but is found wanting or clearly wrong in dealing with other aspects. The availability theory cannot adequately explain the cyclic aspects of drug-abuse epidemics, or why even in areas where abuse is endemic more individuals don't abuse drugs than do, or why with equal availability some individuals use drugs and others don't. The disease theory founders on the inability of psychiatrists and others to agree on a single personality state, or even a group of personality traits, that characterizes most addicts and, more important, that has predictive value. The socioeconomic theorists and the proponents of the social factors tend to overlook the extent of drug abuse in a wide variety of cultures and under widely disparate economic and social circumstances. One is forced to conclude that either we don't know the principal cause of drug abuse or that such abuse is a phenomenon of great variety and complexity explainable by one set of factors in one circumstance and a different, perhaps opposite, set in other circumstances. The role of community mental health becomes somewhat clearer if one adopts this position and argues that the response and remedy must be suited to the particular locale and arrived at only after careful study of the particular problems in that area. Further, because of the complexity of the situation, mental health workers must remain open-minded and modest and aware that even with the best intentions and adequate funding, they may not solve the problem or make even a lasting dent in it.

COMMUNITY INFLUENCE ON DRUG USAGE

The ways in which the actions and attitudes of a community may impinge upon and influence the whole spectrum of drug-taking behavior are summarized in the following list. While some of the factors described may be beyond the ability of local forces to shape, they are mentioned as directions in which the community can try and exert pressure on the state or national government. Not all the factors apply in every community. Nor can one be sure that even if remedies suggested from these points are undertaken, substantial reduction in drug abuse will follow.

1. Community attitudes, often expressed in or manipulated by advertising and the media, can define the kinds of situations in which drug taking is socially acceptable, romantically deviant, or quite abhorrent. Examples of this are numerous but at times subtle. It is easy to spot radio or TV advertisements that show how the schoolteacher who is unable to cope with her noisy class adjusts after taking an over-the-counter tranquilizer (and thus tacitly condones the youngster taking his tranquilizer—marijuana or a barbiturate—to cope with a screaming teacher). Equally obvious is the parent who automatically equates stress or relaxation with the need to take alcohol. More subtle are lectures and articles lumping together all drug use as equally dangerous and unlawful, so that the youngster who takes some pills sees himself as a romantic outlaw whose risk-taking behavior will make him a hero to his peers. From the opposite point, the campaign in which drugs were conceptualized as preventing certain desired community objectives appears to have had some effect on inner-city drug use (e.g., "Wake up, it's Nation Time", "Black Is Beautiful, Black and on Dope Isn't"). Community and peer pressure can be powerful weapons in shaping behavior if the goals of the individual are perceived by him as consonant with or dependent upon community or peer goals and approval. If the girls in a high school define the drug user as "cool" and the nonuser as "square," the incentives for a male adolescent to use are enormously multiplied.

2. The community creates the social, economic, and psychological climate in which the individual finds drugs useful to avoid or cope with one or another facet of that climate. The use of heroin in ghetto communities is often explained as an attempt to blot out the depressing socioeconomic realities of everyday living there. Heroin use in suburban areas may provide both surcease from social and academic competitive pressures and a rationalization for nonachievement in those realms. Psychedelic use in suburbia may be an attempt to fill a spiritual void created by the obsolescence of much of institutional religion and the emphasis on material abundance.

3. By its legal and political machinery, the community defines which drugs people can have ready access to through normal legal channels and which they can acquire only by illegal means. Although such decisions are made at the state and national level, local pressures have a substantial effect. When marijuana use spread to the suburbs, the political pressure generated by parents concerned that their children would go to jail led to reclassification of marijuana possession as a misdemeanor rather than a felony. Similar ongoing pressure has led in many communities to a situation where the police do not make marijuana arrests unless someone lights up in front of them. When heroin use became more widespread in the suburbs, heroin maintenance became talked about more and more and might have occurred in this country if use had not begun to decline.

4. The community can make it easier or more difficult for individuals to obtain

the financial means to get illegal drugs. In affluent areas parents often provide their children with money to purchase drugs out of fear that otherwise they will commit crimes to get the money. In inner-city areas the addict often obtains his funds through the community's willingness to purchase the goods he has stolen, usually from his own community in the first place. Cities affect either way the drug user's financial burden by the rules they set up that determine whether he can get welfare payments.

5. The community can make available adequate funding for preventive and educational programs which may affect the extent or nature of drug taking. In a later section such programs are listed and commented on. Many of them can be seen either as possible alternatives to drug use or as activities that relate generally to the quality of life in a community rather than specifically to drugs.

6. Through the level of resources provided and the emotional climate, the community can encourage or discourage the provision of adequate treatment that might prevent the spread of drug use by contagion from current users. Although substantial funds for treatment now come from the federal government through the National Institute of Mental Health and the Special Action Office for Drug Abuse Prevention, matching funds are usually necessary from the state or community. Certain kinds of programs, e.g., drop-in centers, often find it difficult to get governmental funds or are unwilling to apply because of record-keeping requirements and must depend on local resources. Community attitudes toward certain kinds of treatment approaches, e.g., methadone maintenance, have at times prevented such programs from operating. In other situations communities have approved of the treatment philosophy, e.g., the residential therapeutic community, but have adopted a "not in my neighborhood" stance that has markedly delayed the setting up of such houses.

To the extent that mental health programs can influence the community's behavior in some or all of these areas, they can influence what will happen in a given locale around the drug issue. When they fail to deal with the problems or do so ineffectually, then drug use can help to destroy a community. Criminal behavior by narcotic addicts, for example, can so terrify and demoralize a community that its members either move out or, if that is not possible, remain in a state of fear and resignation amid burned-out buildings. In more affluent areas, drug abuse does not usually present the same degree of physical violence but can similarly render the strivings and goals of parents ineffectual and cause them to despair as they see their children turn to drugs. The fear of drug abuse may drive a community to vigilante action or to support of law-enforcement excesses which violate constitutional standards. The breaking down of doors, smashing of furniture, and harassment of a house's occupants in the name of law enforcement have long been a complaint of inner-city areas. As such raids begin to happen more and more often in middle-class areas—and at wrong addresses to boot—the country may realize the dangers both of drug abuse and of the overreaction to it.[5]

COMMUNITY RESPONSE TO DRUG ABUSE

The preceding discussion has dealt with some of the theoretical issues involved in drug abuse and its interrelations with the community. This section attempts to describe how a community could go about responding to drug abuse from the vantage point of an individual or group of individuals charged with that responsibility for the community.

The first step is to ask a series of questions:

1. What is the size of the particular community? Is it a major metropolitan city? A portion of such a city? A suburban town? On the outskirts of such a city? An essentially rural community? What is the economic makeup of the area? What is the ethnic and racial makeup? Is the program going to be part of a larger network or does it have to be self-contained?

2. What is the target population? What kinds of drug abusers are the particular focus for the community effort? Is one dealing principally with older heroin users or with adolescent ones? Or is the concern chiefly with adolescent poly-drug use or combinations? Where such information does not already exist, techniques such as school surveys and discussions with current and/or ex-addicts, indigenous community leaders, and health professionals may provide crucial information.

3. What is the extent of the problem in the community? Is one dealing with a small, relatively easily defined group or with a variety of groups of different sizes and with different sets of problems?

4. What is the feeling tone in the community about drug abuse? Where are the concerns? Are they primarily directed toward crime and the type of behavior engaged in by addicts in order to support an expensive heroin habit, or is the community primarily concerned because its own youngsters are involved with drugs and it is worried about their future? Are the concerned areas of community and the affected areas of community the same? Are community leaders worried about what is going on in their community or are individuals in the affluent areas worried about "the criminals from the ghetto areas?"

5. What resources already exist in the community that are attempting to cope with the problem? Are there any existing mental health facilities? Has the criminal justice system set up any rehabilitation programs? What is going on in the schools?

6. What are the general facilities of the area? What recreational facilities exist for adolescents and young adults? What mental health services are available for adults, teenagers, and children? How adequate are the schools academically and in the attitudes of the students toward them?

7. What financial resources might be available for programs? Will the money be predominately federal or state? Is there a possibility of funds from local governmental bodies or the local private sector?

The second step has to do with leadership strategy. There have been two major approaches toward organizing and carrying out effective drug programs: the task force approach and the individual leader approach. In the task force approach a group of citizens is appointed by some governmental unit or comes together as a coalition of social agencies and tries to develop a strategy to deal with a drug problem. In the individual leader approach one or two persons who have the energy and inclination to tackle the task develop a drug program and then try to get community backing for carrying on their work.

Each approach has advantages and disadvantages. The task force approach is more likely to ensure citizen participation from diverse groups and in theory at least has a better chance of success. A disadvantage, common to committees in general, is that the result is often pale compromise between competing forces that satisfies no one but is acceptable to everyone. Other disadvantages are the significant delay in actually implementing programs and the fact that, although many people are concerned, all are involved only part-time.

The most important advantage of the individual approach is that it avoids this last problem. One or a few individuals are devoting practically all their time and attention to the drug program and can make decisions as they go along without backtracking to a committee each time for approval. This approach also avoids many of the delay factors, but has the disadvantage of lacking citizen participation and is in danger of not hearing or of overriding opposing points of view, and of failing if the leader chooses to go elsewhere or gets involved in a different area. In spite of these disadvantages it has been my impression in looking over the various drug programs throughout the country that the more successful ones have evolved from the individual leader model or from a task force model in which one individual assumed full-time responsibility for the drug program. Sooner or later, however, the individual leader must develop a community-based task force approach which can give him access to all aspects of the community and thus a broad base of support.

The third consideration has to do with the parent organization or locus of operation. A community mental health center is a logical parent organization for a drug program and such involvement has in fact recently been mandated by law. Since, however, such centers do not exist in many places, an alternative parent organization must be found. In some communities this has been the local health director's office, in others a hospital, in still others a state agency, a community action group, or an antipoverty program. Medical participation in the program is more likely to occur if the parent organization is a mental health center, hospital, or public health director's office. Community action agencies, grass-roots groups, or antipoverty programs are more likely to be close to the community they serve but risk excluding the affluent areas of the community and thus having difficulty in gaining their cooperation.

To sum up, in beginning to deal with a drug problem, certain questions must be asked and answered about the nature and extent of the problem, existing community resources, the nature of the leadership strategy, and the locus of operations. Once these have been answered, the question arises of the best strategies to be employed. These are discussed below under the traditional headings of primary, secondary, and tertiary prevention. Which among the alternative or competing approaches is best for a particular community is usually decided in reference to the answers developed to the questions just raised.

PRIMARY PREVENTION

In this context, primary prevention can be defined as "the prevention of inappropriate drug use and drug abuse in vulnerable populations."[6] The following discussion concerns both parts of the definition: that having to do directly with drugs and that having to do with the vulnerable population. It is important to reiterate that although specific suggestions are presented, their basis is still to a great extent hypothetical. In the current state of our knowledge it is not clear that any technique definitely reduces, let alone eliminates, drug misuse. At this time elimination of drug abuse should probably be set aside as an impossible goal, and instead efforts should be concentrated on aims such as decreasing abuse per se to a minimum, decreasing the use of more dangerous as compared with less dangerous drugs, decreasing the likelihood of adverse reactions to the drug misuse, and improving the functioning capacity of those who do misuse drugs. Even though no current technique can be clearly relied upon to accomplish all these goals, what follows appears to be the most plausible of the current possibilities. Areas covered include drug education, counseling around psychological problems of adolescence, development of an antidrug peer culture, improvement of socioeconomic conditions, provision of alternatives to drug use, the role of advertising and the mass media, and the drug laws.

Drug Education

That drug abuse can be prevented through education has for the past few years been a premise of both government and community response to the drug scene. In many states drug education is as obligatory as the teaching of English or arithmetic. Initially, drug education was mainly done by law-enforcement officials, not only because they were often the only ones in a community experienced and interested in the drug area, but also because it was felt the way to prevent drug use was to scare youngsters away from it. The scare tactics usually involved two main points: (1) severe legal penalties which included not only imprisonment but the blighting of future career once such a criminal record was established, and (2) the dreadful consequences of drug use to mind and body. As drug abuse continued to increase, the law-enforcement scare lecture became old-fashioned and was condemned by clinicians and educators alike. The prime reason given for the failure of the technique was lack of credibility: Suburban youngsters didn't really believe they'd go to jail for long terms; inner-city youngsters often saw jail as inevitable and in any event not particularly condemned by their peer culture; both groups had too many friends or acquaintances who had used drugs without ill effects to believe that "drugs lead you directly to hell without passing go." Compounding the confusion was the inevitable inclusion of marijuana with the stronger drugs, a viewpoint that ensured audience disbelief in the speaker's pronouncements.

The police approach to drug education was succeeded in many places by the ex-addict speaker. The individual was often a graduate or current resident of a therapeutic community such as Daytop or Phoenix House. Looking remarkably healthy, appearing poised and calm even before large audiences, the ex-addict recounted his wayward life, often in intimate detail. The degradations of the drug scene were compared with the beauty of the openness, warmth, and friendship he had found in the therapeutic community. These speakers were usually popular with audiences, were often invited back by student demand, and tended to outshine any mental health professionals or educators who shared the stage with them. So much so that people began to question whether such speakers prevented drug abuse or actually encouraged it unwittingly. No matter how they painted the picture, what usually emerged was a feeling of the excitement of the drug scene. The drug life, in spite of its dangers, or perhaps because of them, seemed often preferable to the humdrum existence of the audience. The outlaw is a recurrent American (if not universal) folk hero; cops and robbers is an exciting game for all ages (witness the TV popularity of such series); and prostitution fantasies occur in many a teenage girl. Even better, one could enjoy the excitement and emerge healthy, poised, articulate, and the center of attention of a large crowd. Addiction, contrary to all the scare stories, was curable. Finally, the description of the therapeutic community in itself was an attraction to many youngsters—and to their parents. Watching the reactions of both age groups to a Saturday night open house at a typical residential facility, one is struck by the frequency of the remark, "I wish I could live in a place like this." The well-advertised warmth and honesty stand in stark contrast to the loneliness, coldness, and deceit of much of everyday life. These concerns led the ex-addict speaker's popularity to wane.

Simultaneous with the ex-addict speaker in some parts of the country, and preceding or succeeding him in others, was the use of the mental health professional or the educator to conduct drug education. Institutes financed by the National Institute of Mental Health or the Office of Education sprang up in various parts of the country to train such individuals. Until recently, however, most had not received much training. Their talks were often accompanied by films (the great majority of which were in 1972 declared either worthless for the purpose or harmful by the National Coordinating Council on Drug Education). Individuals who had undergone training at the specialized institutes were often sold on the value of group techniques in such education. Unfortunately their training was usually enough to convince them of the value of group sessions but insufficient to allow them to conduct it expertly. The training centers did, however, teach factual knowledge about drugs, correct many myths, and when properly run, left their trainees with healthier emotional attitudes and less hysteria about the drug problem.

When these individuals taught by traditional lectures to large groups, they tended to share the fate of the law enforcement lecturers: The audience tended not to listen. Even though they were factually more correct and less apt to use scare tactics, their message tended to be ignored. To get around this, curricula were developed to gradually introduce drug education into the regular school studies. Unfortunately, in spite of the well-thought-out nature of some of these curricula, they were presented by insufficiently trained teachers or by teachers whose emotional attitudes about drug use conflicted with the objective material to be presented.

The questions then arise, Can drug education prevent drug abuse?[8] Have all these methods failed because they were wrong or because the assignment was an impossible one? Initially, one is tempted to feel the task is too hard. Education has not been successful in many other areas where its attempt was to change behavior rather than impart knowledge. The two groups who may be most knowledgeable about drugs tend to have the highest abuse rates—the medical profession and siblings of current users. In spite of this, I feel there are principles and methods that can be of value. They are as follows:

1. The task must be clearly defined. Are we trying to prevent all illicit drug use or just the heavy use of the addict? Can we as a society tolerate drug experimentation? Can we differentiate between drugs with relative degrees of danger? The importance of this point lies in the oft-made observation that a well-run drug education program may decrease the use of the more dangerous drugs such as heroin, LSD, and barbiturates, but at the same time experimentation with marijuana may increase. I believe that in our current state of knowledge, both about prevention and about the effects of marijuana, such an outcome although not ideal is reasonable.

2. Facts alone are insufficient. Many decisions are made on emotional rather than rational grounds. Facts alone, therefore, may be insufficient to cause desired behavioral outcomes even if one could be sure what both the facts and the desired outcome were. In the drug-abuse field both are at times unclear.

3. Many individuals, and especially adolescents, would benefit from seminars and role-playing sessions on coping with peer pressure and the decision-making process. Peer use and peer pressure are probably two of the most crucial variables that determine whether an individual uses drugs, which drugs, and how frequently. Role-playing sessions can help prepare the vulnerable adolescent to cope better with such pressure when it occurs.

4. Seminars, discussions, and rap sessions that deal with common problems of adolescence are probably more valuable than sessions relating strictly to drugs. The more an individual has trouble coping with situations such as peer rejection, relations with the opposite sex, parental discord, and parental drug and/or alcohol use, the more likely he is to use drugs regardless of the extent of his factual knowledge.

5. Any audiovisual materials (or lectures) used should avoid the errors extremely common to the field. As listed by the National Coordinating Council on Drug Education,[9] these include: (a) "... stating that a particular drug *always* causes or *never* causes a certain specific reaction." Instead, it should be conveyed that "the effects of a drug depend on a complex set of variables

that include dosage, method of administration, purpose of administration, frequency of use, mind set and environment." (b) ". . . blaming the drugs themselves for drug-related problems instead of pointing out the influence of non-drug factors." For example, many of the problems associated with heroin addiction, such as hepatitis, stealing, or malnutrition, relate not to the drug but to the illegal aspects and the way of life that flow from it. (c) ". . . advocating a particular rehabilitation model or public law policy which will 'solve' the problem . . . and implying that if one doesn't use a particular drug one will not have problems. Few films convey the message that there is a need for multi-modality approach to treatment, as well as institutional and social reform to prevent a user from backsliding." (d) ". . . focusing on illegal drugs . . . perpetuating the myth that only illegal drugs are misused." (e) ". . . the erroneous misconception that only young people misuse drugs." (f) ". . . classifying drugs inaccurately and, thereby, ascribing erroneous properties and effects to the drug . . . [or] classifying drugs properly but ascribing inaccurate effects to the drugs." (g) ". . . using settings, film techniques, graphics and formats which reinforce inappropriate generalizations and stereotypes about drugs and their effects and drug users."

6. Audiovisual materials should not be used without discussion. Since it is so easy for individuals to misinterpret even material that seems obvious, it is important that audiovisual presentations be followed by discussions that allow clarification, interpretation, and emotional reaction to the material.

Counseling on Problems of Adolescence

Individuals try drugs for many reasons. Among those listed in surveys are curiosity, boredom, peer pressure, peer influence, a desire for kicks or excitement. From individual interviews it is clear that many of these "reasons" are mainly rationalizations.[10] They serve to conceal from others or from oneself the underlying motivations, which may include depression, chronic anxiety, a need to prove one's masculinity, or an attempt to escape external surroundings and circumstances viewed as oppressive and beyond one's ability to cope. Although most youngsters who try drugs, especially marijuana, have no deep-seated problems, it is a safe assumption that those who continue beyond marijuana and beyond experimentation are using drugs to alter either their internal environment or their perception of their external surroundings. Although controlled studies on the subject cannot be cited, it appears a reasonable assumption that helping adolescents cope with the problems cited above as well as with the crises of normal adolescence might diminish the number that progress beyond marijuana and beyond experimentation.

Examples of psychological difficulties with which many adolescents have to cope include rejection by the opposite sex, feeling nonaccepted by one's peer group, constantly quarreling parents, excessive drinking by one or both parents, absence of one parent, and inability to keep up at school especially if one can't read properly. The list could go on and on. It is, in fact, much easier to construct such a list than to devise methods of doing something about the items on it. Considering the numbers of youngsters involved, individual counseling is probably out of the question for all but a very small minority. This, however, may be less of a bane than a blessing, for it seems to me often more appropriate anyway to cope with these areas in a group setting. The group setting provides a number of advantages over the individual approach: The adolescent can learn his problems are not unique to him; interaction with peers may help alleviate a common problem in and of itself; proposed solutions coming from peers may be better received than those emerging from interaction with an authority figure; the participants in the group may be helpful to each other outside of the group. Many of these advantages carry dangers as well and require skill to prevent the dangers from outweighing the possible benefits.

One version of the group approach, the rap session, is being increasingly used in high schools and youth centers. Group leaders include older students, teachers, ex-addicts, and mental health professionals. Mental health centers can play a valuable role in facilitating this possibly preventive tool through encouraging schools in their area to try such approaches, through consultation and training of group leaders, and as manpower resources in providing leaders. Such involvement would provide an opportunity to prevent the enthusiasm for the technique from carrying it to harmful excesses. Poorly trained leaders and failure to recognize and refer especially troubled students are common dangers.

Development of an Antidrug Peer Culture

One of the remarkable changes that occurred between the 1950s and the 1960s was in the attitude of high-school students toward those in their school who used drugs. In the 1950s such students were treated as social pariahs; by the late 1960s they had become cultural heroes, they were cool and daring, not chicken or square. In some places using drugs was a quicker way to gain peer recognition and status than social, athletic, or academic achievement. One cannot say exactly how much this attitudinal change caused (as opposed to followed) the rapid rise in drug use in the 1960s, but my experience in Connecticut schools indicates some of the possibilities. Youngsters wavering about drugs pressured into use for fear of being considered out of it; youngsters on the social periphery using drugs to prove their manliness and daring with the hope of thus becoming accepted; youngsters pretending to drug use and effects to avoid being called chicken. The banana-peel-smoking fad of the late 1960s—part hoax on the Establishment, part reality to many engaged in it—is a beautiful example of how youngsters got high or pretended to get high on an innocuous substance they believed others were getting high on.

If the peer group has such influence on the actions of teenagers, then a logical preventive measure is to develop an antidrug peer culture. Such a culture could provide support to youngsters who don't want to use drugs in the first place, provide acceptance for those who would use drugs mainly to avoid feeling left out, and disseminate information about drugs more acceptably and believably than could adults. Formation of such a culture is, of course, difficult. In the Far West, the

Smart Teens Movement achieved some success. In some inner-city areas community groups appealing to racial pride have been able to turn around groups in some schools. In New Haven we tried assigning some staff and residents of our adolescent therapeutic community on a full-time basis to a local high school. Their charge was to work with non-drug-using teens and develop a number of activities including rap groups, recreational activities, and a variety of work groups centering around interests of the students. Initially, 15 students were involved in the center, which had its own room in the school, and the hope was to expand using the initial students as leaders for new activities and new students. Currently the project is in limbo, a result of unresolved and essentially petty conflicts with the school hierarchy and some poor choices on our part of personnel who did not have the consulting skills to resolve the differences. Although the idea still appears a good one, it clearly requires more attention from high-level and skilled mental health personnel than we had been willing to devote to it.

Improvement of Socioeconomic Conditions

Certain addicting drugs, especially heroin, have tended to be used in a chronic and sporadically epidemic fashion in areas of socioeconomic deprivation in our major cities. This has occurred regardless of who was in these ghetto areas at the time—the immigrants of the 1920s or the blacks and Puerto Ricans of the 1940s, 1950s, and 1960s. Many observers felt that the way to decrease heroin use in those areas was to improve socioeconomic conditions. Heroin was seen as a response to the depressing social conditions surrounding the individual and as a way of escaping such conditions by decreasing awareness of them. While most reasonable persons agree on the necessity and desirability of improving conditions in these deprived areas, there is less consensus that such improvement would indeed lead to decreased heroin usage. One possibility is that as socioeconomic conditions improve drug use per se may not change but the type of drug used may change. And since the type may change from more harmful to less harmful drugs, the end product may be a lessening of overall drug abuse. Therefore, it seems logical that as one attempt at primary prevention, mental health programs should lend their support to efforts to improve housing, employment, education, and other areas of life that tend to produce a chronic despair in many ghetto residents. Such efforts can take place though working with community leaders, through direct action with the resources that mental health programs have at their command, and through political pressure on various government bodies.

Provision of Alternatives to Drug Use

Anyone who has lectured frequently to audiences on the subject of drug abuse is likely to have been asked, Why do adolescents use drugs? What many adults do not realize is that this is typically an adult question. The adolescent is more likely to ask, Why not? As mentioned earlier in the chapter, the usual responses to the latter question have to do with variants of fear—fear of the law, fear of the physical or psychological effects of the drug, or fear of the consequences if significant others (e.g., parents) find out about the drug use. As the number of youngsters using drugs increased and it became clear that negative approaches were not working, more attention was paid to the possibility of positive alternatives to drug use. The subject has still not received as much space as it deserves, but some recent articles have been encouraging.

Underlying the alternative approach is the assumption that drugs are used for a reason and that providing a non-chemical method of achieving something similar may be sufficient to keep the individual away from chemical means. Since there are numerous reasons behind individuals' drug use, no single alternative can be a panacea. A group wishing to diminish drug abuse must contemplate providing a variety of alternatives. In one recent article,[11] for example, 11 different groups of possible reasons for drug use are cited and possible alternatives to each of these listed. The 11 groups are physical, sensory, emotional, interpersonal, social, political, intellectual, creative-aesthetic, philosophical, spiritual-mystical, and miscellaneous. Possible motives in each of these categories are given and corresponding alternatives are likewise cited. Some have already been mentioned in this chapter: use of counseling to handle psychological problems; use of rap groups to deal with the everyday concerns of adolescents. Rather than repeat all the alternatives described, it seems more useful to consider three general principles that should be kept in mind when trying this approach. First, the alternative should be active rather than passive. Second, the alternative should be incompatible with drug use. As is pointed out in the article just cited, listening to music may be a useful alternative in the sensory sphere, but not unless it precludes being stoned while listening. Techniques or ways of listening would need to be taught so that being stoned would interfere with the experience, not enhance it. Third, it is important to realize that expressed motives and underlying motives may not be identical.

The alternative method appears to work best with nonusers and experimenters. With the heavy user or drug-dependent individual, it is often necessary initially to enforce the alternative of "not using" before more positive alternatives can be suggested. Mental health programs can aid school systems in developing alternatives as part of the curricula or as extracurricular activities. In the former situation it is probably preferable to offer them in a nongraded manner. The community as a whole can also be helped to consider what alternatives can be developed on a communitywide basis. A community that offers few recreational and social facilities for its teenagers and young adults has little grounds for complaints when these individuals hang around street corners and doorways and take drugs for recreation. Finally, mental health programs would be well advised to consider how training in nonchemical alternatives could be implemented in their own work with individuals and groups.

Role of Advertising and the Mass Media

There has been a great deal of publicity concerning the effects of publicity on drug use. Traditionally, this has taken the form of criticism of the advertising of mood-altering, over-the-counter drugs. Recently, however, antidrug commercials and general stories about drugs have come under fire. Unfortunately, there has been much more rhetoric on both sides than actual documentation of what effects such publicity has. The few existing studies were reviewed in the second report of the National Commission on Marijuana and Drug Abuse.[12] They suggest that, while advertising alone may have relatively little influence compared with family and friends, it may serve to reduce internal conflicts by implying to users that everyone turns on in his own way. One of the studies cited also suggested that users of illegal drugs tend to be more receptive to pharmaceutical advertisements than nonusers. While the commission was against government intervention in this area, it did recommend that the media on their own initiative reexamine the impact of informational messages on youthful interest in psychoactive drugs. In connection with such reexamination it recommended that the media sponsor and support longitudinal research into the effects of various communications on behavior. Further, the commission felt that, with respect to proprietary mood-altering drugs, no advertising should suggest that the substance can result in pleasurable mood alteration or alleviate malaise caused by stress or anxiety.

The role of mental health professionals in this regard can be as follows:

1. They should pay attention to the way substances are advertised in their community, in the press, radio, or television. If they feel the advertising is too suggestive, they should make their views known to the media owners. In Connecticut, for example, the drug subcommittee of the Connecticut Conference of Mayors has taken the initiative in monitoring certain television stations and calling to the attention of the stations involved those advertisements which seem too suggestive of the need to use chemicals to cope with everyday anxiety.
2. In any statements or articles done by the media in the community, mental health professionals should be careful that material is not sensationalized. As an example, articles dealing with methaqualone abuse which display the fact that it is called "the love pill" and is seen by some teenagers as an aphrodisiac are more likely to stimulate interest than any of the details in the story about its dangers are likely to discourage interest.
3. Centers should do their best to cooperate with or initiate research projects which may provide more facts in this area so that we do not have to continue relying on guesses, no matter how informed.

Drug Laws

Social control of drug use relates to two areas: public attitudes and the legal system. Prior to the Harrison Act in 1914, control depended mainly on public attitudes; in the 60 years following that legislation the legal system provided the chief instrument.[13] Depending on the time period and the drug involved, different segments of the public either supported or ridiculed the various control mechanisms. Legal prohibitions against heroin availability, for example, have tended over this period to reflect the opinion of the overwhelming majority of the populace, while those against alcohol in the 1920s and marijuana currently have found large segments of the public opposed.[14] In situations where this polarity occurs, the issue becomes political and enforcement is erratic and may reflect factors other than concern about drug use per se (e.g., hirsute teenagers are more likely to be arrested for marijuana use than conservatively dressed businessmen).

This state of affairs leads some to argue that the ". . . law really is the major cause of the drug controversy."[15] If the laws governing possession, use, and perhaps even sale were dropped, they insist, not only would more effective social controls emerge but the current costs of such laws—alienation; diversion of scarce police, judicial, and correctional resources; and corruption of law-enforcement agents—would be eliminated. The legal controls would be replaced by education, treatment, rehabilitation, and a value system believed in and acted upon by the people.

The difficulty with this position is that while it would offer improvement in some areas of our current drug difficulty, historical precedent suggests that it would create other problems. The numbers using potent drugs irresponsibly would increase, and the corrective forces suggested at best would take a long time to emerge and at worst might not emerge in any viable form at all.

The position can be understood, however, as a response to the frustration created by the drug laws in existence today. While the frustration is real and justifiable, improving the laws is a better solution than discarding all of them. Drugs should be classified on the basis of medical rather than legal judgment, penalties for violation of laws pertaining to possession or sale should relate to the dangers of the particular drugs involved. It would be foolish to solve our marijuana problem, however, by worsening our heroin and barbiturate problem. In a number of states, the pressure of mental health groups and concerned citizens has led to better laws; in some states, however, the laws remain a nightmare. To argue that some laws are necessary does not mean that the other areas cited are not also necessary. Social control of any behavior is most effective when the majority of the populace supports the aim of the control and when there is a unifying value system. The success of China currently in solving its drug problem appears to be a combination of very harsh drug laws and a social ethic and value system subscribed to by the majority.[16] One would guess that if this ethic is weakened, China's drug problem would again increase.

SECONDARY PREVENTION

Secondary prevention in the drug area "seeks to stop drug abuse in an individual before he has become addicted or become identified with a drug abusing and addicted subculture."[6] There are two groups at risk in this context: those persons who have begun to experiment with drugs or who use them on an occasional basis, and those who have not begun to use drugs but who, because of the existence of certain problems (relating to families, the law, their school, or their interpersonal relations), seem likely eventually to get into serious difficulties with drugs. In addition, certain community practices relating to and supportive of drug abuse are discussed below as part of secondary prevention.

Helping the Individual at Risk

Available evidence, both clinical and survey, indicates that the majority of individuals who experiment with drugs such as marijuana stops at the experimenting or occasional use level.[12] The same appears to hold true for most individuals involved with solvent inhaling. A number in each group, however (and estimates range from about 5 to 15 percent), become involved with more dangerous drugs. This more extensive involvement may relate to peer pressure, an attempt to handle certain personal or social problems, or a conscious choice of a certain way of life and life style. The suggestions offered below relate to material touched on in the sections on drug education and alternatives to drug use, since the line between primary and secondary prevention in the drug field is a thin one.

COMMUNITY RESOURCES CENTERS

These centers could be established in both inner-city and suburban areas with the components of each center determined by the needs and characteristics of the particular population to be served. It is important that representatives of such populations be involved in the planning. The following are some basic services that such centers might offer.

Recreational facilities. These not only attract adolescents and young adults to the centers but also serve as a useful way for individuals to spend leisure time. Although it was commonly believed some years back that athletics and drugs didn't mix, that if an individual got involved in sports he would not get involved in drugs, there have been many exceptions. Furthermore, there have been enough stories and exposés from the sports world demonstrating the at times extensive use of a variety of drugs by both professional and amateur athletes to refute any simple notion that the two don't mix. These facts do not preclude the possibility that recreational activities can help some youngsters avoid drug use. It has been my observation that one of the main problems drug-dependent individuals have is an inability to use leisure time in a satisfying way. The individual who is trying to stay off drugs finds most difficulty during evenings and weekends. Not only does he have more free time then, but he does not know what to do with the time. Therefore, recreational facilities should be planned with an eye toward involving individuals in group activities and providing training in recreational activities that can be used later in life. Recreation is, of course, not limited to athletics, and these facilities should provide or be able to arrange for individuals to enjoy a variety of artistic pursuits. The more active these pursuits, the better. Although passive recreation may supply a way of initially attracting certain parts of the population, it is better to have individuals involved in making movies than simply watching movies.

Rap sessions. The centers should offer the opportunity for rap sessions and seminars, enabling individuals to discuss in a general way problems common to their age group. Training in peer-group counseling, human relation skills, and communication skills could also be made available at the centers.

Individual and group counseling. Often clients for this service identify themselves to the center's staff after rap sessions or seminars, or they may be identified by the staff because of the way they relate to others during such sessions or during the recreational activities. Where possible, peer-group counseling should be emphasized. Mental health professionals should be available as backup and as consultants to the essentially indigenous or paraprofessional staff of the centers. It would be useful if medical backup were available for those cases where unwanted pregnancies and venereal disease, to cite two examples, are involved. Along with the general counseling function of the center, staff should be trained in crisis-intervention methods.

Education. Since diplomas are an increasingly important part of our current society, it is essential that staff and volunteers at the center be sensitive to problems youngsters may be having in school—difficulties of an academic nature or with peer group or with teachers. The center, perhaps with the use of volunteers, could provide some tutoring for academic difficulties and the previously mentioned functions for the interpersonal difficulties. At times, it may be useful for the center to work with other groups in the community to develop educational alternatives such as street academies and free schools. For a youngster who has already dropped out of school, the staff should work quickly to use peer pressure to get him back into an academic setting or into job training.

Reaching-out. Individuals who come to the center should be encouraged to get involved with their community in working on whatever they identify as pressing problems in that community. In one area this might take the form of ecological projects; in another it might consist of using older teenagers as big brothers for fatherless younger teenagers. An additional kind of reaching-out is to encourage the youth as well as the staff to attract to the center other individuals in the community who might benefit from it. Such centers often miss the youngsters who most need them, and these youths can be more successfully reached by their peers than by staff. It is important also that the center not be identified as a drug center. Although seminars about various aspects of drugs can be part of the center's activities, this should not be emphasized as it is more likely to turn off youngsters than to attract them. Drugs should be seen as one of the areas that adolescents are interested in, just as they are interested in individuals of the opposite sex, in peer relations in general, in local and national problems, and in what they are going to do in the future.

GROUP HOMES

Many adolescents regularly come to the attention of health, mental health, other social agencies, or criminal justice agencies, to whom it is clear that the behavior they are engaged in or the problems they present are going to be difficult,

if not impossible, to deal with as long as they remain in the same milieu. Currently, there are relatively few alternatives for housing youths. The traditional state
reform school or correctional center for adolescents has been aptly characterized
as breeding more crimes than it prevents, and to avoid drug dependence and delinquency among this group alternatives to these institutional placements must be
found. One possibility is the residential youth center. Such a center, usually holding from 7 to no more than 20 individuals, located in the community, and staffed
by young adults with professional backup, can be an important alternative placement that removes the youngster from his disturbed environment and keeps him
out of an equally disturbing correctional institution. The small size, family atmosphere, staff-youth interaction, and community setting make such homes preferable
to the large, isolated correctional setting. Ironically, they can also be cheaper. In
Connecticut, for example, the yearly expenditure per youth for such homes is
$6000 to $8000 compared with $14,000 to $19,000 for the large training
schools.[17]

Two types of facilities in this category can be conceptualized: the group home
model where the youngster stays for a prolonged period, and the crisis center
model where he stays for a few days up to a few months while the immediate
family crisis is resolved and from which he can return to his family.

Tacit Community Support of Illicit Drug Use

In this context I am not talking about peer-group support for certain drug use
but rather the means by which the community furnishes the background for continued illegal activities by which addicts support their habits. Most heroin addicts,
for example, at one time or another, resort to property crime to get money for
drugs. Items are stolen from stores or private homes and then sold "on the
streets." While certain items are disposed of through professional fences, most go
directly to the individuals who will use them. This market enables lower-income
individuals to have access to radios, television sets, automobile accessories, clothing, at prices far below retail cost. It also ensures the addict a ready market for
his stolen wares and thus money for his habit. While it is easy to condemn this
lower-class version of the middle-class "I can get it for you wholesale," it clearly
fills a social need that is fueled by the consumption ethic and advertising practices.
While it is probable that if addicts quit stealing, enough economically marginal
individuals exist to keep thieving alive, the volume of theft would probably be
smaller without the drive of the heroin addict behind it. Even though many of the
stolen goods come from the same neighborhoods in which they are being sold, it
is unlikely that the practice will cease until there is an improvement in the socioeconomic status of these communities.

Intensive Outreach and Treatment

To the extent that drug abuse follows a contagious disease model, early intervention and treatment directed at areas where a sudden increase is noted may have
striking effects.[18,19] To be successful, such intervention should be preceded by

epidemiological field investigations and pilot outreach and treatment efforts. The fieldwork can assess the size of the outbreak, the location, and the characteristics of those involved. The pilot outreach and treatment efforts can help gauge whether the treatment offered is going to be attractive to the population in question and provides an opportunity to hire and train indigenous personnel who can then attract others from the same area. These initial efforts should be followed by intensive outreach and treatment; then, even when numbers begin to decline, persistent efforts should be maintained to work with new cases, old ones who have relapsed, or those who resisted treatment initially. Since this model relies heavily on voluntary admission to the program, the support of community leaders and organizations, and treatment programs seen as desirable by the drug users, are all necessary.

TERTIARY PREVENTION

Tertiary prevention "aims to treat individuals who are addicted to drugs (or involved heavily in subcultures of drug abuse) in such a way as to control the disability and facilitate psychological and social rehabilitation."[6] Given the limits of our current methods, it is likely that many individuals so treated will have some degree of residual disability and that a number will from time to time relapse to active drug involvement. In this sense then drug dependence is similar to other chronic medical disorders, both psychological and physical. In the late 1960s there was a tendency to romanticize addicts, to believe they were individuals with enormous talents which would be released once they stopped putting all their energies into procuring and using drugs. In retrospect this illusion appears to have sprung from two sources: the significant success of many early therapeutic communities and methadone programs, and the skill addicts were able to display in their hustling careers. Mental health professionals and other members of the community kept believing that if this energy and talent were turned to positive pursuits, the results would be tremendous. Reflection indicates that the early successes were not repeated consistently and that a substantial number of narcotic addicts, even when no longer taking drugs, have residual psychological as well as social difficulties.

The type, duration, and effectiveness of treatment are greatly influenced by the individual's psychological and social assets and liabilities. Regardless of the claims of various treatment programs, no one method is effective for all or even most patients, and the same individual may need different kinds of treatments at different stages in his drug-using career. Not only is there a lack of agreement about the various treatment approaches, there is disagreement about what the goals of therapy are. The two most common goals are cessation of drug dependence and social rehabilitation. Different schools of thought give varying weights to the two objectives. For some, a program which involves maintenance, e.g., by methadone, is ipso facto not treatment because dependence on a drug is continued. Others consider the key goals to be employment and lack of criminality, and argue that if these can be achieved, legal drug use or occasional illegal drug use is unimportant. Regardless of which goals are espoused, there is disagreement over the effectiveness of the various approaches. Proponents of the different treatment methods talk about success rates between 60 and 90 percent, while critics cite figures of between 10 and 50 percent.[20,21] Part of the disagreement arises from different methods of counting. For example, if 90 percent of the graduates from a therapeutic community are doing well, but only 50 percent of the individuals entering such a program graduate, is the success rate 90 or 50 or 45 percent? A second reason for disagreement arises from the issue of goals. Is treatment successful if the patient remains on a methadone program, or only if he is on such a program and urinalysis shows no use of illegal drugs, or only if he is employed, or only if he gets off of methadone, or all of these? Depending on which criterion is chosen, success may be 70–80 percent (retention rate), 40–80 percent (clean urine), 35–75 percent (employment), 20–60 percent (all the factors). In short, statements about success can be misleading unless the criteria for success are clear. Generally, current treatments especially for narcotic users appear much more successful than those available prior to the 1960s. For nonnarcotic drug users, however, fewer methods are available and these are not as effective. Balancing this is the clinical observation that users of nonnarcotic drugs are usually more apt to stop drug use on their own than are narcotic addicts, who remain on their drug for long periods, until they "mature out."

Since there are good descriptions of the various treatment approaches already in the literature,[6,20,22] this chapter does not attempt to cover the subject comprehensively. Instead, a few comments are noted on each method to indicate some of the existing problems. The principal treatment modalities are outlined below. Whereas in the 1960s they tended to operate as separate entities, the preference in the 1970s has been toward multimodality, toward a central program offering a number of different options.

A. Maintenance
    1. Narcotic maintenance
        a. Methadone
        b. Heroin
        c. Combinations or other narcotics
    2. Narcotic antagonists
        a. Naloxone
        b. Cyclazocine
        c. Naltrexone or other new agents
B. Abstinence
    1. Self-help therapeutic community
    2. Traditional psychotherapy, inpatient or outpatient
    3. Drop-in centers
    4. Religion-oriented programs
    5. Behavioral conditioning
    6. Experimental approaches

The maintenance approaches at this time are confined to the treatment of narcotic addiction, although it is possible that at some time in the future chemicals of the antagonist variety will be available for treatment of sedative and stimulant dependence. The abstinence approaches can be used for the treatment of drug abuse in general, regardless of the particular drug involved.

Methadone Maintenance

Methadone maintenance involves the use of a daily basis of a synthetic narcotic, methadone, as a replacement for heroin. At the usual dose range (50–100 mg once daily) it reduces or eliminates drug-seeking behavior, blocks the effects of the average street amount of heroin, permits the individual to function without undue drowsiness or euphoria, and has a minimum of other side effects. Since its introduction in 1964, it has become both the most widely used treatment for heroin addicts and one of the most controversial. Debated questions include the following:[23] What degree of ancillary supports—psychotherapy, vocational counseling, etc.—should be given with the methadone? How long must maintenance be continued? Can or should individuals be weaned from methadone or should they take it indefinitely? If methadone eliminates drug craving, why do so many methadone users continue to take narcotics? Is the risk of diversion to the illegal market worth the gains produced by maintenance? Does a maintenance approach put too much power into the hands of those running the programs?

The methadone approach has the distinction of being attacked by both poles of the political spectrum. On the right it is attacked by some because of the fear of diversion and by others who view any maintenance of addicts as immoral per se; on the left its attackers see it as a plot by the Establishment to control the lives of minority people.[6] Unfortunately, all these attacks have tended to obscure the central fact that has emerged after 9 years of use of the drug for maintenance. This can be stated as follows: Given in a well-run program, methadone maintenance enables a significant number of program participants to function as productive human beings without use of other drugs and without criminal activity. It is clearly not the ideal treatment, since the individual remains dependent upon a drug and withdrawal of that drug can be difficult. Some of the problems associated with methadone maintenance arise from ambiguities about why it is used. Clinicians tend to see it as a way of removing the patient from his psychological dependence on the chemically induced high state and drug-seeking way of life. Whether it is also necessary clinically to treat a "metabolic craving" induced by being addicted is debatable.[24] Society at large, however, often views methadone maintenance as principally a way of decreasing the crime necessary to support a drug habit. Where this view predominates, programs may become simply "dispensing stations" and, ironically, there may be much less impact on crime, since the other factors associated with criminal behavior by addicts are not dealt with.

Heroin Maintenance

Heroin maintenance is not used in the United States, though many individuals and groups have urged that it be given at least a limited trial. As available in England, it has been called the medical distributive model—providing the addict with the drug of his choice under medical auspices. It is based on the idea that narcotic addiction cannot be successfully treated in many cases and providing the drug in an inexpensive pure form is the best alternative for the individual and society. Whether the system which has worked reasonably well in England could be transplanted here with our greatly different social problems and already developed illicit market is the major unanswered question around which controversy rages. Other important questions include: Would providing heroin maintenance discourage the use of other treatment methods which have a better chance of leading ultimately to abstinence? Would heroin maintenance make addiction less fearful and more acceptable and thus entice more teenagers? Can individuals on heroin maintenance assume socially productive roles?[25] Although the evidence from England tends to favor our trying such an approach on a limited scale,[26] there is such emotional feeling on the subject that it is doubtful whether such an experiment will soon occur. This is especially so since the current heroin epidemic appears to have peaked and numbers of users are markedly declining. Forgetting social and emotional factors, heroin maintenance from a medical point of view is not as good as methadone maintenance for three reasons: heroin is not very effective by mouth, necessitating several injections daily; it is relatively short acting, requiring two to four doses every 24 hours as compared with one for methadone; and it produces a much greater degree of euphoria than oral methadone and could thus interfere with social rehabilitation.

Narcotic Antagonists

These agents have been known for quite a while but only recently have been used in an ongoing maintenance approach. They may eventually become the most important chemotherapeutic approach for narcotic addicts, replacing methadone maintenance. Like methadone they block the effects of heroin. Not only does the individual not feel the euphoria of the heroin but additionally he cannot become physically addicted even if he takes the narcotic daily. Unlike methadone, the antagonists are not themselves physically addicting and, therefore, eliminate the problem of eventual withdrawal that has plagued methadone programs. When an individual first starts on antagonists he must be narcotic-free, since one of their other actions is to precipitate immediate withdrawal symptoms if the individual is addicted. There is controversy in the literature over whether individuals maintained on antagonists should be encouraged to try narcotics or discouraged. Those arguing the first point of view do so from a conditioning model of addiction.[27] With that model it would of course be important that the individual try narcotics so that the conditioned response he previously experienced be extinguished. The other approach, which is the one we have used in New Haven, holds that the individual is best treated by getting him out of the drug life and if he periodically takes narcotics and is associated with a narcotic-using group he will likely discontinue the use of the antagonist.[28]

The mechanics of an antagonist maintenance program are relatively simple. Once the patient is free from narcotics, he is started on a small dose of the antagonist which is gradually increased until stabilization is achieved. The final dose reflects the amount of narcotic to be blocked, the duration of action, and certain side effects. The antagonist effect is a quantitative one and like the methadone blockade can be overriden by taking very large quantities of narcotics. Although theoretically possible, for the most part such overriding is economically difficult and usually does not occur.

Three antagonists that have had some clinical trials are cyclazocine,[29] naloxone, [28,30] and naltrexone. Cyclazocine has been used for a longer time and has the advantages of lasting from 24 to 28 hours in the usual clinical dose. Unfortunately, however, during the induction phase especially, there are some unpleasant side effects which for many patients has made taking the drug an unpleasant experience and therefore decreased their willingness to be involved in such a program. Since such side effects can be blocked with naloxone, it may be possible to interest more patients in using this drug. Naloxone has far fewer side effects than cyclazocine but has the disadvantage of a shorter duration of action. In the usual clinical dose it only lasts about 18 hours. Naltrexone, which is the newest of the antagonists to be tried clinically, is a chemical combination of the other two drugs. In the trials so far it appears to have the duration of action of cyclazocine with the minimal side effects of naloxone and overall appears to be well tolerated by patients at the usual clinical dose.[31,32] Experiments are going on now to increase the duration of action of naltrexone by increasing the dose and to develop new antagonists with longer duration of action. In addition research is in progress on depot preparations which would involve giving an antagonist in a form that could last from 2 to 4 weeks, or even longer. Having used all three antagonists in the New Haven program, it is my feeling to date that naltrexone is the best of the three. Since these antagonists only block the effects of narcotics, they must be used in the context of various kinds of psychosocial support. If the addict's social and psychological problems are not dealt with, even though he may not be able to use narcotics, he's likely to get high on something else which could be even more destructive. In short, the antagonists to be most effective must be given in a regimen that treats the person rather than simply the particular drug of dependence.

Even if new long-acting antagonists are developed they may not achieve the popularity of methadone. The difficulty concerns consumer acceptance. Even though the individual stabilized on methadone does not get high from that drug, he experiences to some extent a relief of drug craving. Since this does not occur with the antagonists, it will be interesting to see whether patients will volunteer to take them as readily as they volunteered to take methadone. From a community mental health point of view the antagonists have a potential which is both promising and frightening: Since they can block addiction without being themselves addicting, there is a strong possibility that they will be considered for preventive purposes for individuals who have never been addicted. While such a concept has some similarities to water fluoridation and smallpox vaccination, it raises a host of civil liberty issues which cannot be easily dismissed. Since the technology for such a project is not more that a few years away, concerned groups must begin to think out the possibilities so that we do not come upon them unawares as has been the situation with so many other scientific developments.

Detoxification

Once considered treatment in and of itself, most programs now regard withdrawal from drugs as only the first step in treatment or even as pretreatment. Withdrawal from narcotics even without medical help can be painful but should not have a fatal outcome.[23] Through methadone substitution and withdrawal, detoxification becomes a relatively simple procedure which can be carried out on either an outpatient or inpatient basis. Withdrawal from barbiturates, on the other hand, can be a life-threatening process and should be carried out on an inpatient basis. Abrupt cessation of amphetamines may lead to severe depression and suicide, and therefore should also be done on an inpatient basis. Panic reactions related to drugs such as LSD can be treated on an outpatient basis with tranquilizers, or, even better, the individual can be talked down, as is usually done at crisis centers. In all these cases the problem is not treatment of the withdrawal state, which is fairly readily done, but prevention of the chronic relapsing condition.

Self-Help Residential Therapeutic Communities

Since Synanon, the prototype of the therapeutic community for treating drug addicts opened in California in the late 1950s, many similar houses have opened across the country. These descendants differ from Synanon in their emphasis on individuals eventually returning to the community as opposed to remaining in Synanon as part of a permanent subculture. They differ from each other in factors such as length of stay (6 months to 2 years), degree of educational and vocational counseling input, use of some professional as opposed to all ex-addict staff, and amount of deviant behavior tolerated. There are, however, far more similarities than differences. These include emphasis on confrontation group therapy; a relatively rigid hierarchical structure; a reward and punishment system based on a fairly strict value code which emphasizes honesty, openness, a family feeling, and taking of responsibility, and forbids violence or drug use. A marked advantage of these communities is that, unlike methadone, they are open to drug users regardless of the drug of abuse. As heroin use subsides somewhat and youngsters turn increasingly to sedatives and stimulants, the ability to treat polydrug users will be a pronounced asset.

The major problem of these programs concerns retention rates.[20] It has become increasingly clear that these programs are not for everyone. Even though it appears that most of their graduates do well, losses prior to graduation may range from 50 to 90 percent of all who enter. Since the programs already are rather selective in terms of admission, improvement of retention rates may have to depend more on internal changes than improved selection. A second problem has to do with reentry. A frequent complaint directed at these programs is that graduates tend to end up working in the same or other drug programs rather than in more diverse occupations. A third problem concerns whether the current philosophy of these houses is so middle-class oriented that they cannot effectively reach individuals from socioeconomic strata that do not share these values.

Traditional Psychotherapy

Psychiatric inpatient and outpatient programs appear to be helpful mainly with two kinds of individuals: the older, more middle-class person who had demonstrated some ego strength and job stability prior to using drugs; and the adolescent user who has not been taking drugs long enough to develop many of the secondary characteristics of drug addiction and for whom drug use has not become the most important aspect of his life. For these two groups the pure psychiatric approach seems to have some merit. For others, it appears to have none. One of the reasons for this on the inpatient units may be the "we-they" problem. If the setting is a traditional psychiatric unit, there are the patients and the staff, and the barriers are hard to break down. Because of the two different cultures, the staff members often do not know about the sub rosa activities of the patients. If one thinks of drug addiction as a character disorder, and argues that the way to change character disorders is to intervene as quickly as possible after the occurrence of the behavior that should be changed, the sine qua non is to know that that behavior has occurred. If staff members do not know until a week later, because of a conspiracy of silence among the patients, the staff cannot intervene in a way that will effectively change behavior. The self-help residential centers are much less prone to this kind of difficulty.

Group therapy often is more effective than traditional one-to-one psychotherapy both because of the peer pressure that can be exerted on the user and because the group can more effectively cut through many of the denials, rationalizations, and manipulations employed by the patient. Individual therapy, however, can be useful after the individual has stopped using drugs. It has been my experience that graduates of therapeutic communities are often excellent candidates for such an individual approach.

Drop-In Centers

The drop-in or crisis center is one of the commonest drug programs found across the country. Staffing and direction range from all adolescents to mixtures involving adolescents, young adults, adult volunteers such as parents, teachers, and clergy, and mental health professionals. At times the centers are primarily directed toward drug users, but more often they are involved in a whole variety of problems including depression, running away from home, venereal disease, and unwanted pregnancy. Some stress activities such as music and art, while others emphasize individual counseling or rap sessions. Some see themselves as treatment centers, while others are primarily interested in consciousness raising and may be more interested in helping adolescents use drugs more safely than in pursuading them to total abstinence.

For the most part these centers have worked with psychedelic and amphetamine users and have referred narcotic addicts to other programs. Those that have tried to reach addicts often find that the relatively loose structure of the program cannot handle the manipulations of the confirmed user. With the recent turning away from heroin among adolescents and the substitute of barbiturates and amphetamines, these centers may have increasing importance. Unlike some of the programs previously described, which usually require full-time involvement, these centers offer a splendid opportunity for mental health professionals to work in a significant and yet part-time manner either as consultants to lay staff or as a direct source of manpower.

Religion-Oriented Programs

There is a wide spectrum of religion-oriented groups and programs. One of the oldest is Teen Challenge, a residential program started in Brooklyn in the late 1950s which now has 40 centers throughout the country. The program has a number of distinct differences from the self-help programs, and these differences are useful to understand the nature of the program.[20]

1. Unlike the self-help houses, the program avoids confrontation techniques as exemplified in the encounter groups. The workers feel that these techniques break down individuals who are already broken, and instead they emphasize supportive approaches that stress an individual's goodness.
2. Instead of the emphasis on work and group therapy, a resident's time may be spent in prayer, Bible study courses, speaking in churches, and street work with addicts.
3. Religious conversion is expected of the residents, although not necessarily to a specific denomination.
4. Greater emphasis is placed on family counseling and reconciling the individual with his family.

5.   In addition to illegal drugs, residents are expected to give up cigarettes and alcohol.

There are no reliable statistics about the outcome of the Teen Challenge programs. Although glowing reports are given of their successes, it appears that the percentage of graduates is no greater than, and probably less than, programs such as Daytop. The program in the East appears to be particularly attractive to Puerto Rican addicts and in the West to Mexican American addicts. Women addicts tend to do poorly and not to remain in the program.

Closely related to the Teen Challenge program is the Jesus Movement (at times known as Jesus Freaks). Although loosely defined and differing from place to place, the program does seem to have certain differences from Teen Challenge:

1.   It is less likely to be residential in nature.
2.   Members are more likely to be middle-class psychedelic users than minority group heroin addicts.
3.   Rapid religious conversion is again the norm but with less rigorous studies demanded, less follow-through, and greater claims of success (often over 90 percent). These success claims have not been objectively studied and are probably at least 80 percent too high.

At another point on the religious spectrum one finds an emphasis on Eastern rather than Western religions or at times attempts to combine the two. The most popular variant is Transcendental Meditation, an approach which has attracted thousands of individuals, most of whom are not drug users. The vast majority of drug-using individuals trying this approach are the psychedelic and amphetamine users rather than heroin addicts, and no follow-up has been done to see whether favorable results last over time. Transcendental Meditation has the advantage of being able to be done alone without the aid of a program once the technique has been learned. The individual, through the meditation, is supposed to be more relaxed, self-confident, energetic and yet not frenzied, and able to tap his inner resources.

Another religious approach is that of the Black Muslims. This group, a variant of the Muslim religion (the traditional Muslim religion does not involve a black-white dichotomy), appears to be a combination of religious, racial, and nationalistic ideas. It is said to be effective (again not documented objectively) among older black heroin addicts, but has had much less success in attracting and holding (as have had most other drug programs) adolescent addicts.

A common denominator between the religious and the self-help programs is the fervor with which their adherents view their programs and their tendency to vehemently put down other approaches, especially those involving maintenance. This intolerance has at times had unfortunate consequences, as when the political power of the Phoenix House approach in New York City kept that city, the birthplace of methadone maintenance, lagging behind the rest of the country in applying methadone maintenance on a scale commensurate with the number of addicts to be reached. There are hopeful signs that this parochialism is changing toward a recognition that, given the diversity of addicts, it is necessary to have a multiplicity of approaches.

Behavioral Conditioning

Although a number of the programs already described are based to a greater or lesser extent on principles of behavioral modification, they do not involve the kind of rigorous experimental structure that is formally known as behavioral conditioning. As practiced in the treatment of drug dependence, this in the past usually involved negative conditioning—the pairing of what has been viewed as pleasurable (e.g., the injection of the drug) with painful or unpleasant stimuli (e.g., an electric needle which gives shocks or administration of a nausea-producing drug concomitant with the narcotic).

Some of the more recent behavioral approaches have involved attempts at positive reinforcement using variants of a token economy. Unfortunately, there are few reinforcers that can rival the immediate pleasurable aspects of the substances they are trying to condition addicts not to use.

Experimental Approaches

In addition to the programs already described are a variety of techniques which can be loosely grouped together as experimental approaches. None of them have been used extensively in the treatment of drug-dependent individuals, and so far they do not appear to be the rapid, miraculous type of treatment that enthusiastic proponents have at times pictured them. Periodically a new variety of experimental approach makes headlines briefly only to prove disappointing after further trials.

CARBON DIOXIDE INHALATION THERAPY

This has been used with mixed results for over a decade in the treatment of a wide variety of psychiatric disorders. Its adherents are enthusiastic, others are skeptical. A recent attempt in Philadelphia to treat narcotic addicts with carbon dioxide was suspended following the death of two patients which may or may not have been related to the treatment.[34] The treatment consists of the patient's breathing pure oxygen for a minute or so, then inhaling 75 percent carbon dioxide until he passes out—in approximately 45 seconds. Finally, the patient is revived with 100 percent oxygen. It is claimed that two such treatments a day will detoxify heroin addicts with no withdrawal symptoms, and by taking the treatment periodically after that, the addict will remain off heroin.[35]

LSD THERAPY

Long before LSD became a drug of abuse and widely used by adolescents, it was tried by mental health professionals as therapy for a variety of psychiatric conditions. The two main variants of this form of therapy were psychedelic and psycholytic. In the former, after some preparation concerning what the experiences would be like, the patient was given a large dose of LSD, usually 250 μg. The drug experience took place in a variety of settings designed to elicit a psychedelic experience. This, plus the follow-up work by the therapist, were the main components of the treatment. In the psycholytic approach, the patient was given a smaller dose of LSD and an attempt was made to conduct therapy while the person was under the influence of the drug. In this context the drug was being used to decrease the resistances and defenses of the patient to permit certain material to emerge that could then be worked on in therapy.

LSD therapy has been used rather extensively in the treatment of alcoholism and on a much more limited basis in the treatment of drug dependency.[36] The enthusiastic claims of success for such treatment are not borne out by follow-up studies,[37] and except in a few places, such therapy is no longer being carried out.

ALPHA-WAVE CONDITIONING

The alpha wave is a normal component of an individual's brain waves. During electroencephalographic monitoring alpha waves appear when the individual is in a relaxed state which, upon questioning, he will define as pleasurable. It is interesting to note in this connection that when an individual is given heroin, alpha waves predominate for the first 15 minutes or so. In a process known as biofeedback conditioning, in which the individual learns to produce certain changes in his body by receiving instant feedback about the results of his efforts, individuals can be taught to produce alpha waves at will.

Claims for the beneficial effects of alpha wave have included increased relaxation, increased creativity, decreased difficulty in falling asleep and remaining asleep, and in general, a state of meditative relaxation that has been called a drug high without drugs. Alpha-wave conditioning is becoming increasingly popular among adolescents and young adults, especially thsoe involved with psychedelics. Although the theory is promising, it is too early to say how useful such an approach will be in the overall treatment of drug dependence.

CONCLUSION

While drug abuse may be mainly a disease of the spirit, it carries with it possibilities of serious harm to the individual, his immediate social environment, and the larger community. Our difficulty in being able neither to cope with it nor accept it in a rational fashion illustrates our inadequate knowledge of the phenomenon and our failure to act adequately in those areas where there is some understanding. To the extent that it is influenced by a variety of community attitudes and behavior, the preceding material, which suggests some actions that can be taken, may be a useful starting or review point for individuals involved in community mental health. We must remember, however, that the desire to alter one's state of consciousness is a strong one and that drug use is seen as a quicker and easier way to achieve this than most alternatives. At best, therefore, society's efforts are likely to ameliorate the situation rather than prevent it. It appears very human to believe that the grass on the other side of the hill is greener. It is but a short step for many to act on the proposition that grass makes the other side of the hill seem greener.

REFERENCES

1. Eddy NB, Halbach H, Isbell H, Seevers MH: Drug dependence: Its significance and characteristics. Bull WHO 32:721–733, 1965
2. Frosch WA: Psychoanalytic evaluation of addiction and habituation. J Am Psychoanal Assoc 18:209–218, 1970
3. Chein I, Gerald DL, Lee RS, Rosenfeld E: The Road to H: Narcotics, Delinquency, and Social Policy. New York, Basic Books, 1964
4. Gay AC, Gay GR: Evolution of a drug culture in a decade of mendacity. In Smith DE, Gay GR (eds): It's So Good, Don't Even Try it Once: Heroin in Perspective. Englewood Cliffs, NJ, Prentice-Hall, 1972
5. Malcolm AH: Violent drug raids against the innocent found widespread. New York Times, June 25, 1973
6. Meyer RE: Guide to Drug Rehabilitation: A Public Health Approach. Boston, Beacon Press, 1972
8. Halleck S: The great drug education hoax. Progressive 34:30–33, 1970
9. Drug Abuse Films (3rd ed). An evaluation report by the National Coordinating Council on Drug Education, Washington, DC, 1972
10. Kleber HD: Student use of hallucinogens. J Am Coll Health Assoc 14:109–117, 1965
11. Cohen AY: The journey beyond trips: Alternatives to drugs. In Smith DE, Gay GR (eds): It's So Good, Don't Even Try It Once: Heroin in Perspective. Englewood Cliffs, NJ; Prentice-Hall, 1972
12. Drug use in America: Problem in perspective. Second report of the National Commission on Marihuana and Drug Abuse. Washington, DC, GPO, 1973
13. Musto DF: The American Disease: Origins of Narcotic Control. New Haven, Yale University Press, 1973
14. Kaplan J: Marijuana: The New Prohibition. Cleveland, World Publishing, 1970
15. Roberston JA: The drug laws: Problems of overcriminalization. In Brown CC, Savage C (eds): The Drug Abuse Controversy. Baltimore, National Educational Consultants, 1971
16. Lowinger P: How the Chinese solved their drug problem. Med Opinion 2:81–92, 1973
17. Judging youth correction homes (editorial). New Haven Register, June 26, 1973
18. Hughes PH, Crawford GA: A contagious disease model for researching and intervening in heroin epidemics. Arch Gen Psychiatry 27:149–155, 1972
19. Hughes PH, Senay EC, Parker R: The medical management of a heroin epidemic. Arch Gen Psychiatry 27:585–591, 1972
20. Glasscote R, Sussex JN, Jaffee JH, Ball J, Brill L: The Treatment of Drug Abuse: Programs, Problems, Prospects. Washington, DC, Joint Information Service of the American Psychiatric Association, 1972
21. Maddux JF, Bowden CL: Critique of success with methadone maintenance. Am J Psychiatry 129:440–446, 1972
22. Kleber HD: The treatment of drug dependence. In Edwards R (ed): Current Considerations in Drug Education. Englewood Cliffs, NJ, Prentice-Hall (in press)
23. Kleber HD, Klerman GL: Current issues in methadone treatment of heroin dependence. Med Care 9:379–382, 1971
24. Dole VP, Nyswander ME: Heroin addic-

tion: A metabolic disease. Arch Intern Med 120:19–24, 1967

25. Lewis E Jr: A heroin maintenance program in the United States. JAMA 223:539–546, 1973

26. Kramer JC: Controlling narcotics in America. Drug Forum 1:153–167, 1972

27. Wikler A: Some implications of conditioning therapy for problems of drug abuse. Behav Sci 16:92–97, 1971

28. Kleber HD: Clinical experiences with narcotic antagonists. In Fisher S, Freedman A M (eds): Opiate Addiction: Origins and Treatment. Washington, DC, Winston, 1973, pp 211–220

29. Freedman AM, Fink M, Sharoff R, Zaks A: Clinical studies of cyclazocine in the treatment of narcotic addiction. Am J Psychiatry 124:57–62, 1968

30. Zaks A, Jones T, Fink M, Freedman AM: Naloxone treatment of opiate dependence: A progress report. JAMA 215:2108–2110, 1971

31. Martin WR, Jasinski DR, Mansky PA: Naltrexone: An antagonist for the treatment of heroin dependence. Arch Gen Psychiatry 28:784–791, 1973

32. Resnick R: Personal communication

33. Glaser FB, Ball JC: Death due to withdrawal from narcotics. In Ball JC, Chambers CD (eds): The Epidemiology of Opiate Addiction in the United States. Springfield, Ill, Thomas, 1970

34. Death puts a sudden halt to CO_2 therapy for drug addicts. Med World News 14:36–37, 1972

35. Can CO_2 smother heroin addiction? Med World News 14:5, 1972

36. Savage C, McCabe OL: Residential psychedelic (LSD) therapy for the narcotic addict. Arch Gen Psychiatry 28:808–814, 1973

37. Ludwig AM, Levine J, Stark LH: LSD and Alcoholism: A Clinical Study of Treatment Efficacy. Springfield, Ill, Thomas, 1970

Morris E. Chafetz, M.D.

8

Alcoholism

Nine million Americans suffer from a chronic, disabling, and potentially lethal disease. The condition cripples their on-the-job performance, or keeps them away from work altogether, enough to cost their employers or themselves $10 billion a year. The victims of this malady cause unmeasured suffering to 40 million other persons, who are close to them. What is more, substantial numbers of sufferers from this disease commit suicide, while many others kill innocent persons, sometimes by intentional homicide, sometimes by "accident." Two thirds of the victims of this disease can be treated successfully, and, if not "cured," at least helped to live reasonably "normal" and productive lives. Yet many in acute stages of illness are turned away by physicians and hospitals, and fewer than 10 percent of the 9 million are under treatment.

The disease, of course, is alcoholism. The data are from the National Institute on Alcohol Abuse and Alcoholism (NIAAA).[1] It is fair to say that alcoholism is the most frequently untreated treatable disease in America today.

HISTORY AND ATTITUDES

In part, that sad fact is due to our ambivalent attitude toward alcohol, a drug which has played an important role in this country since the rum trade was a mainstay of the colonial economy. Whisky offered the frontiersman one of the three generally available avenues to momentary forgetfulness of the hard, dangerous, and dirty meanness of his life. (The other two are mentioned in the line from the west-

---

The views expressed here are those of Dr. Chafetz speaking in his private capacity and do not necessarily represent those of the Government.

ern folk song, *Streets of Laredo,* describing the cowboy's payday: "First down
to Rosie's, and then to the card house . . .")

The bragging buckaroo who could out-do his fellows at everything else often
tried to outdrink them, as well. The very fame of skid row which does not exist,
is a remnant of the Paul Bunyan days.* In the cities, male immigrants, without
the restraint of family ties, were also tempted to seek comfort in the bottle. Succeeding waves of immigration brought us people of different cultures, many of
whom used alcohol in different ways and had low incidences of alcoholism, for
example, Jews who use wine on ceremonial occasions and Italians who drink it
almost exclusively at meals. Yet many of their descendants appear to have adopted
the American pattern. Studies have shown that Irish-Americans drink more than
the Irish in Ireland and that third generation Italians have higher rates of alcoholism than did their grandparents.[2–4]

Paralleling this stream of history, however, was another that also ran strongly,
the Temperance movement, of which Carrie Nation, swinging her axe in saloons,
provides us with such a vivid picture. The Temperance people viewed alcohol as
the Demon Rum and the drinker as a willful sinner whose inevitable course was
a quick slide to total degradation. True temperance did not exist; the only way
Hell could be avoided was through total abstinence. Young Temperance women
really meant it when they said, "Lips that touch liquor shall never touch mine."
Their ultimate triumph was, of course, Prohibition.

One consequence of our history is that 64 percent of Americans still think
it is at least partially true that "alcoholism is basically a sign of moral
weakness."[5] Thus, while the use of alcohol is widely accepted, there is often
an inner sense that the act of drinking it is somehow wrong, even sinful; guilt feelings frequently accompany drinking.

Another consequence is the popular tendency to think of the alcoholic person
in terms of the skid row bum, still clutching his muscatel bottle as he passes out
on the sidewalk in a pool of vomit; he is paying the ultimate price in degradation
for his "sins." In fact, such people constitute only between 3 and 5 percent of
our alcoholic population. It is far harder for many people to think that the alcoholic person may be the salesman who needs his three martinis before lunch "to get
through the afternoon," the factory worker who does not take a drink all week
but who goes on a blinding Saturday night binge, or the suburban housewife who
nips away the day from a bottle in the kitchen cabinet. Alcoholism is bad, goes
the feeling, and these people are too much like oneself to be bad. In fact, according to NIAAA, "About 70 percent or more of the alcoholic population consists
of men and women who are still married, still holding a job—often an important
one—and still are accepted and reasonably respected members of their communities. For those of this group who seek treatment, the outlook is quite
optimistic."[1] Yet the stigma that remains upon the name "alcoholic" is such

---

*The name is a corruption of Skid Road, which was a long, steep street in Seattle, so called because
new-cut logs were skidded down it from the hilltops to the sawmills at water level. The street was solidly
lined with saloons and brothels.

that many doctors will not treat alcoholic patients; half of our more than 7000 general hospitals will not accept them under that diagnosis.

The popular movement to win recognition for alcoholism as a treatable disease is relatively new, and may be said to have begun when Alcoholics Anonymous began to receive wide publicity in the early 1940s. In the historic *Driver* and *Easter* decisions of 1966 and in *Powell vs. Texas* in 1968, the Federal courts established the disease concept in law. The law sadly needed reforming; nearly half of all the 5 million arrests per year in this country are made for alcohol-related offenses, such as "public intoxication" and "vagrancy." A long step forward was taken in 1971 when the National Conference of Commissioners on Uniform State Laws agreed upon a model Uniform Alcoholism and Intoxication Treatment Act, which included a policy statement that "alcoholics and intoxicated persons may not be subject to criminal prosecution because of their consumption of alcoholic beverages, but rather should be afforded a continuum of treatment in order that they may lead normal lives as productive members of society." On the Federal level, the great forward leap was made when the Congress enacted the Comprehensive Alcohol Abuse and Alcoholism Prevention, Treatment and Rehabilitation Act of 1970, creating NIAAA and requiring the states, as a condition for receiving Federal grants, to set up comprehensive alcoholism plans. All 50 have now done so.

A DEFINITION AND ITS IMPLICATIONS

A commonly quoted definition is, "An alcoholic is anybody who drinks more than I do." Though this is said jokingly, it reflects the important truth that a person's attitude toward his own drinking may deeply influence his attitude toward the alcoholic person. To a Prohibitionist, the statement may be taken literally to apply to a person whose only imbibing is a glass of wine with dinner. To a physician who is maintaining tight control over his own drinking, the consumption of more by someone else may well seem excessive, even in the absence of other symptoms, because he knows that such amounts would be dangerous for him. At the same time, he may close his eyes to obvious symptoms in someone who drinks *less* than he does because to diagnose such a patient as alcoholic is to threaten his own self-evaluation.

A definition adopted by the World Health Organization is

Alcoholism is a chronic behavioral disorder manifested by repeated drinking of alcoholic beverages in excess of the dietary and social uses of the community and to an extent that interferes with the drinker's health or his social or economic function.[6]

However, this more serious definition also lends itself to subjective bias (what is excess in what "community" and who says so?). It also concerns itself more with group deviance than with the individual and focuses on the late stages of the disease.

Chafetz and Demone preferred this definition:

We define alcoholism as a chronic behavioral disorder which is manifested by undue preoccupation with alcohol to the detriment of physical and mental health, by loss of control when drinking has begun (although it may not be carried to the point of intoxication), and by a self-destructive attitude in dealing with personal relationships and life situations.[7]

By focusing on *preoccupation*, we avoid the subjective question of "community standards." "Loss of control" refers to both psychological and physiological responses. The self-destructive element is very important. If the patient cannot function or deal with everyday frustrations without dependence on alcohol, he needs help, whether or not he is violating community norms.

Using this definition, it becomes clear that there is no single "alcoholic personality," but that alcohol problems can and do occur in all types, and that alcoholism is actually but one element in a whole complex of psychological, social, and physical disturbances. In one sense, indeed, alcoholism may be seen as a manifestation of underlying problems which the drinker is unable to deal with in more constructive ways. If a man's wife has left him, if he has been fired, or has just been evicted, he is hardly likely to stop drinking until he can see some better way to deal with those circumstances. It is of little help to him to point out that drinking caused all of this in the first place; the patient is far more acutely aware of that than the physician is. He suffers an enormous burden of guilt for just that reason; that is why he seeks bottled oblivion.

This is why it cannot be too strongly emphasized that treatment must be tailored to the individual. There is no broad-spectrum antibiotic for alcohol-related problems. Each person being different from all others, each with his or her own personal problems, treatment must be tailored to the particular self and set of problems. Perhaps the greatest single cause of failure in the treatment of alcoholism has been the insistence of practitioners and agencies upon playing Procrustes: if the traveler did not fit the innkeeper's preconceived bed of treatment, then he had to be either shortened or stretched until he did so. The only other alternative was to turn him away from the inn altogether, blaming him for lack of what used to be called "willpower" but today is more fashionably referred to as "motivation." What was forgotten is that preset programs may not motivate people; help with their problems, as they *perceive* them, does.

Because the range of problems that may underlie or relate to an alcoholic person's drinking is so vast, an equally comprehensive range of services needs to be available. This requirement goes far beyond such elemental things as the supply of food, lodging, and a set of clean clothes to the skid row bum. An employed person may need hernia repair or surgical correction of an eye defect to keep on working; an unemployed one may require vocational counseling. The person may need legal advice to get him out of a scrape or financial counseling to deal with an overwhelming mountain of debt. He and his family may need various social services.

Simple referral of an alcoholic person to an agency that may help with one of his problems, however, is not enough. Fragmented care too often turns out to mean no care at all. Any person who has had experience with the multiclinic out-patient department of a large hospital is only too well aware that simple shuffling even nonalcoholic patients from one office to another results in a most disheartening drop-out rate. A study at the Massachusetts General Hospital describes some of the barriers that formerly discouraged alcoholic patients there, and shows that the elimination of barriers and decrease in waiting time spectacularly increases patient response.[8] An alcoholic person who cannot handle the problems he already has is hardly the person to take on new frustrations.

Fortunately, there are other ways. One person, to whom the patient relates warmly and who will see to it that the promised help is actually delivered, can be in charge. The H. Douglas Singer Zone Center, a state facility at Rockford, Ill., has firmly written agreements with 16 different agencies and no patient sent to any of them under its agreement may be turned away. Control is also maintained within the Center itself.[9] Similarly, because it is the whole person who is to be cared for, it is preferable that an alcoholism unit not stand in isolation, but rather that it be an ordinary part of a comprehensive center in a health or social agency setting where multiple facilities are available and where the alcoholic person is treated just as is any other patient.

PREVENTION AND EDUCATION

The vast majority of Americans who drink do so pleasurably, moderately, responsibly, and without harm to themselves or others. Episodes of excess, if they occur at all, are rare and not likely to be repeated. There is no evidence whatever that even lifelong use of alcohol in this fashion is harmful. But what works for most people obviously does not work for all. Thus the decision whether or not to use alcohol is a personal one, to be made by each individual. Those who do choose to drink, however, assume a responsibility not to harm either themselves or others by reason of that choice. The responsible use of alcohol can, and has been, successfully taught for many hundreds of years as, for example, in the Italian family whose children learn early that wine is a pleasant adjunct to meals, but that drunkenness is socially unacceptable conduct.

If the national epidemic of alcoholism is to be brought under control, treatment and rehabilitation efforts must be broadened and intensified, but the great weight of our long-range hopes must rest upon prevention and education. Even if every diagnosed alcoholic person were "cured" tomorrow, the flow of new patients would not stop. We will have to do no less than change the attitudes and practices of a large segment of American society. We know by bitter experience that Prohibition and the preaching of total abstinence simply do not work for a great many people. Hence, the inculcation of a sense of responsibility must be the key—responsibility, not only in the initial decision to drink, but in the whole series of decisions that flow from that one—what to drink, how much, when, and under what circumstances. In short, the individual must be able to fit the use of alcohol safely into his life pattern and if excess occurs or other problems arise, he must be able to reevaluate and perhaps modify his behavior. Obviously, this requires not only that he be acquainted with the facts about alcohol but that he absorb them in sufficient depth to provide motivation and influence conduct. *Education* must have occurred, and most education does not occur in schools.

A preventive campaign should disseminate the facts—both positive and negative—about alcohol, patterns of problem drinking, and alcoholism. It should also promote self-awareness among both drinkers and nondrinkers, encouraging them to *think* about drinking, to be conscious of peer and social pressures and to learn how to handle them. Among principles that should be recognized are that it is not essential to drink; many a former problem drinker has learned how to ask for ginger ale without spoiling the party, and the thoughtful host will keep his glass filled with just that. Heavy drinking is not a mark of manliness, nor is drunkenness something to be laughed at. Alcoholism is not a sin, but it is the signal of a troubled person in need of help. Drinking does not help emotional problems; alcohol cannot improve (rather it is quite likely to worsen) the reality of a situation; it only momentarily alters one's perception of that situation.

It is important that individuals learn the effects of alcohol upon themselves, for example that the average person will metabolize the drug at the uniform rate of about 1 oz/hr, with variations according to body weight and food consumed at the time. Thus, for most people, drinking no more than a jigger of whisky or a 5-oz glass of wine or a pint of beer per hour will not permit alcohol to accumulate in the blood. The importance of body weight should be made especially clear to small people. Sometimes "a good little man" will try to stand up drink for drink with an imbiber twice his size. He usually loses.

A drinker should learn that his psychological and physiological condition, as well as the social context in which he drinks, will influence his reactions to the drug. The drinker also must recognize the effect his drinking may have upon his obligation to others; his drinking pattern should be one that he would want his children to emulate (because they probably will), it should neither cause nor aggravate marital conflict, nor should it embarrass others on social occasions. Most emphatically, of course, he should recognize the dangers of driving after drinking.

The drinker should also be made aware that some commonly used drugs—even ordinarily safe ones—have an additive or potentiating effect with alcohol. Additive means that the drug simply adds its effects to that of the alcohol. A potentiating or synergistic drug does more. When it is taken with alcohol, the effect of *each* is heightened; the total effect is increased geometrically, so to speak, rather than arithmetically. Barbiturates are synergistic with alcohol; the combination can be, and often has been, lethal. Tranquilizers are also potentiating. The stronger ones, such as chlorpromazine (Thorazine) or prochlorperazine (Compazine) can be dangerous, even in small amounts, if taken without medical supervision. The minor ones, such as meprobamate (Miltown) and chlordiazepoxide (Librium) are also potentiating with alcohol. Taken with liquor, they can cause unusual drowsiness, endangering anyone who is, for example, operating machinery or driving a car. Even the antihistamines, which are sold over the counter in cold remedies, motion sickness medications and the like, are additive with alcohol and can cause life-threatening drowsiness.

A fundamental aim of an educational program should be to develop in the individual a strong self-respect. Armed with that, he can develop his sense of responsibility towards others. Upon reflection on these points, it will be seen that "alcohol education" is "about" a great deal more than alcohol. It is, in fact, an integral part of education for living, for meeting the demands that are placed upon one, and, like much other learning, it only begins in the schools.

It is obvious that all of this involves a great deal more than giving an annual illustrated lecture in the schools. The subject must be integrated throughout the school curriculum, wherever appropriate, and there are a great many appropriate places besides the course on "hygiene," for example, times when the school is planning a major social event. A teacher who looks over his or her school with that point in mind will have little difficulty in finding other occasions. It is vital, however, that what is taught relate to the actual experience of the pupils if it is to be accepted. A great many teenagers experiment with alcohol at a much younger age than some elders may suspect, and a few do more than experiment. Need we recall again that Prohibition does not work? It is far better that early experimentation be controlled and channeled into a healthy direction.

The most important influence over the child, however, is the model that is set for him at home. An in-school program should thus be only a part, albeit an important one, of an integrated program covering the whole community.

Prevention and education programs are now being operated by many diverse groups—medical societies, hospitals, community centers, industries and businesses, civic groups. The Junior Chamber of Commerce, through its local chapters, is supporting an effort on a national scale, using materials and assistance supplied by NIAAA and by the American Hospital Association and working closely with existing local groups and state agencies. A promising beginning has been made, but much more is needed.

EARLY DETECTION AND DIAGNOSIS

All too often, a problem drinker has to "hit bottom" before a diagnosis of alcoholism is made and treatment begun. In part, this is because the medical profession shares the layman's ambivalent attitude toward alcoholism. Blane, et al. found that even well-trained, well-motivated young physicians were captives of the skid row stereotype. Even when symptoms pointed toward a diagnosis of alcoholism, they tended not to make that diagnosis in patients who had a medical or surgical condition on which they could focus, who were married, employed. had medical insurance, and had not been brought in drunk by the police.[10] Thus an alcoholic person who is "respectable" may be allowed to continue on his self-destructive way, rather than being offered help at a time when treatment is most likely to be successful.

In 1972, the National Council on Alcoholism published a set of diagnostic criteria in order to provide the physician with objective standards.[11] The NCA criteria separate symptoms into two "tracks." Track I lists those that are physiological and clinical; Track II, those that are behavioral, psychological, and attitudinal. The manifestations are further classified as early, middle and late, major and minor, and weighted for diagnostic importance.

Three diagnostic levels are given numerical values. Those persons who meet criteria weighted as Number 1 are said to have a definite diagnosis of alcoholism. Levels 2 and 3 are indicative and should arouse suspicion, but diagnosis should be confirmed with additional evidence. If any of the major criteria are present in one track, the physician should look for symptoms in the other.

Level 1 criteria include on the one track such symptoms as a blood alcohol level of more than 150 mg/100 ml without gross signs of intoxication, withdrawal seizures (differentiated from seizures due to other causes), alcoholic hepatitis, and delirium tremens; on the other track, drinking despite medical contraindications known to the patient and drinking despite strong social contraindications (such as job loss or arrest for drunken driving). Level 2 signs include blackouts, fatty degeneration in the absence of other known cause, and the patient's complaint of loss of control, while Level 3 signs include such things as flushed face, nocturnal diaphoresis, SGOT elevation, the choice of employment that facilities drinking, and major family disruptions. If only minor criteria such as alcoholic facies, tachycardia, or drinking to relieve anger are present, *several* criteria in both the physical and behavioral tracks are necessary for diagnosis.

These criteria represent an important contribution in that they further clarify the parameters of the illness. However, they continue to focus on late stages. Much too little is known about the progression from early problems to the classic late stages of alcoholism.

Imperfect though the diagnostic art be, danger flags fly early in the game. The NIAAA notes that any of the following may indicate an alcohol problem: gulping drinks to hurry the effect; starting the day with a drink; drinking alone because of boredom, loneliness, or to escape reality; drinking behavior that causes either family or job problems; rationalizing drinking behavior; frequently overindulging; blackouts; drinking to relieve hangovers; requiring medical attention as a result of drinking; or frequent minor accidents or physical complaints.[12] Physicians often overlook such signs. If the patient presents with a treatable physical complaint, the doctor may simply concentrate on that and not even ask the questions that will give him a clue as to what is really going on. A check for the early signs of an alcohol problem should be as routine in his practice as a check for the early signs of hypertension.

Those who would detect the early signs should give particular attention to members of high-risk groups, such as persons whose parents were alcoholic persons. It has long been observed that alcoholism tends to run in families. Various studies have indicated that a male relative of an alcoholic person runs a three to six times greater risk of becoming an alcoholic person than does the general population. Using the figures from these studies, Amark noted that it would appear that one of every four first-degree male relatives of a male alcoholic individual will also be an alcoholic individual.[13] The progression may not always be from father to son. A son may react so strongly against his alcoholic father as to become a rigid teetotaler with total abhorrence of all drinking by anyone (in itself an unhealthy form of preoccupation). His own son, in turn, may react equally against his father's repression and follow his grandfather's pattern. And, although the evidence remains inconclusive, some recent studies indicate that genetic factors may play a role in familial alcoholism.[14-16]

Several studies and surveys have pinpointed other social, cultural, and psychological variables that appear to be related to risk. Ethnic background is believed to be a factor. Some investigators have reported that the physical effects of alcohol are markedly different upon American Indians and certain Orientals than they are upon Caucasians.[17, 18]

People who had generally unhappy childhoods or who were from broken homes are also believed to be at higher risk, as are those who grew up in families that had an ambivalent attitude toward alcohol. Religion also may play a part: non-churchgoers, Catholics, and liberal Protestants have a higher percentage of heavy drinkers than do members of fundamentalist Protestant denominations and Jews. Heavy drinkers *and abstainers* were found to be somewhat more alienated and unhappy than moderate drinkers.[2-4]

An optimistic finding is that a "turn over" pattern seems to exist. Some as they grow older, particularly those in the upper middle class, tend to outgrow their problems and are able to return to acceptable drinking patterns. Why this should be true of some people, and not of others, is not understood.

The picture of the high-risk woman is not as clear. A man who is out in the world will have difficulty in concealing a severe drinking problem, but a woman may be protected from exposure for years within the four walls of her home. Thus, one cannot know whether what seems to be a rising rate of alcoholism among women is in fact one, or whether the fact is just that more women are seeking help. Cahalan et al. did find that women are catching up with men in the percentages who drink at least occasionally. However, there was a marked difference in other aspects of their drinking practices. For example, although problem drinking generally first shows up in men who are in their 20s, it does not usually appear in women until they are in their 30s and 40s.[2-4] Like men, some women have outgrown the condition by their 50s.

It is by no means only the physician who should be alert to the early signs and aware of the high-risk potential of certain people and situations. Other professionals and paraprofessionals often see the afflicted person before the doctor does. The troubled person may first visit a clergyman or marriage counselor. A vocational counselor or even an employment agency may be able to spot symptoms. The private practitioner's patient may complain about his hangover within hearing of the office receptionist but not tell the doctor himself about it. The nurse or aide in the hospital may observe things that need not go into the chart but that should be called to the physician's attention. In short, there is a wide circle of people who can assist in early detection if only they are made aware of what to look for and what to do about it.

Industry is playing an increasingly important role in early detection. About 4.5 million workers suffer from alcohol-related problems, and more and more enlightened employers are realizing what this costs them. The special, structured characteristics of the work world make an ideal environment both for identification of persons with problems (through job performance and behavior) and for motivating them to seek treatment (if they want to stay on the payroll). This was recognized as early as 1940 by a few corporations, but early programs usually identified only workers who were in the later stages of alcoholism and whose conditions were too obvious to be concealed any longer. Supervisors were uncomfortable at being asked to diagnose a disease that they felt was basically a matter of character deficiency or moral weakness; some would sympathetically "cover up" for the troubled employee as long as they could. The National Council on Alcoholism sought to apply new research findings to develop new programs during the 1960s, but progress was slow because of the stigma surrounding the employee identified as an alcoholic person. Only a few programs were effective, but of the employees who were reached through them, up to two of every three who accepted treatment remained on the job or returned rehabilitated.

The NIAAA's Occupational Alcoholism Branch surveyed programs across the country in an attempt to find common threads of policy and procedure that identified a maximum number of employees adversely affected by alcohol and that resulted in a high rate of recovery. A major key to success was found to be a clear definition of the role of a supervisor. Alcoholism, even in its earliest stages, results in an alteration of the employee's job performance and his behavior. Other disturbances may also produce changes; it is the supervisor's role, not to diagnose, but only to observe that the work of any troubled employee is suffering and to refer him to a company counseling or assistance service. That service should try to find out exactly what is causing the trouble and put the employee on a course of action designed to deal with his problem. In about half the cases, that problem will be alcohol-related. *Confidentiality must be assured.* The "carrot and stick" approach of combining sympathy for the employee as a human being with firmness about his work generates a powerful incentive.

ORGANIZING A COMMUNITY PROGRAM

In every community of any size there are numerous institutions and individuals who come into professional contact with alcohol problems. The hospital emergency department, the social work and welfare agencies, police, Veterans Administration, physicians, clergymen, educators, employers, visiting nurses—the list of those who see alcoholic people and their troubled families is almost endless.

Unless there is a well-thought-out, clearly organized system, however, the end result is likely to be frustrating on all sides. The client's name may be in the files
of half a dozen agencies, and, yet, he may not be really known to any of them.
Such "shopping around" by patients may irritate agency personnel, but it may
also be a sign that the person himself is trying, however ineptly, to coordinate the
services he knows he needs. It may be that everything he needs is there, if only
he were able to get at it, or there may be gaps that need filling.

In either event, the first step is obviously an inventory of existing resources
within the community to be served. This needs to be more than a mere listing of
agencies and facilities whose programs may exist more on paper than in actuality.
There should be a close examination of what each actually *does*, who is in charge
of doing it, how well it is being done, and for whom it is done. Putting this information together into an organization chart should reveal whether any new services
are needed or whether any reorganization is desirable.

Services provided should include: (a) detoxification centers in hospitals, closely linked with (b) an evaluation and outpatient service, which will provide for
diagnosis of the long-term problem and referral, and which also accepts patients
from all other sources, including the police, and walk-ins; (c) an inpatient center
to provide aftercare in the subacute stage, extensive evaluation and referral for
long-term care; (d) temporary residential care for those who require it and are not
in an acute condition, plus appropriate services; (e) halfway houses and, of course,
(f) long-term treatment. We repeat that provision should be made for one person
to take responsibility for guiding the patient to these and other services that he may
need and for following him up.

Close contact among agencies is obviously required. People may attend each
other's working meetings to become acquainted with each other's possibilities and
plan common efforts; case conferences may be held on patients of mutual interest;
in some instances it may even be possible to make joint staff appointments. Firm
understandings must be reached so that patients do not "fall between the cracks."
Entry to the system at any one point must mean entry to all points.

It is important that planning by no means be restricted to the involved professionals. Strong input from "consumers," in this case, recovered patients who are
familiar with the system from the inside, is necessary. It is also vital to enlist the
cooperation and assistance of outsiders, such as civic groups, service clubs, and
political leaders, whose aid may be required for such matters as raising funds and
obtaining the support of local government. A publicity campaign, both to win general public support and to spread the word of the availability of help is also important. (One study showed that only 44 percent of people know of any place in their
communities where help for alcoholism could be found.[5])

The community will need to inventory its resources of trained personnel.
Treating the alcoholic person requires specialized knowledge and skills which may
be acquired either through formal courses or on-the-job training. Some communities may be "growing their own" quite well; others may need assistance. NIAAA
sponsors training programs for a range of people from recovered alcoholic individ-

uals to medical school professors. In addition, the National Center on Alcohol Education of the NIAAA supplies materials that may be used in training programs. As of early 1974, there were about 100 training programs for all types of personnel scattered across the country.

There are numerous potential sources of funding for community programs in addition to the public campaigns that private agencies may conduct. Support will be easier to obtain if the alcoholism program is integrated into the comprehensive health care delivery system. Consultation with Federal and State agencies, and with local government people, will uncover numerous potential sources of revenue.

Participation of the community and consumer must not be mere tokenism; these people must be *listened* to. The primary loyalty of personnel must not be to the agency that pays their salaries, but to the communities for whom they work. All who work or participate in an agency's functions should share in what goes on there; for example, staff patients, and clients should have some knowledge of the budget, its size, and where it goes and why. Volunteer groups should be encouraged and their efforts utilized. As has been said, "There is no need for defensiveness when criticism is just. The goal is to learn from criticism. And, it should always be remembered, it is impossible to teach, to persuade or to treat others effectively until one's own house is in order."[8]

TREATMENT

Detoxification treatment lies beyond the scope of this chapter. However, it cannot be emphasized too strongly that the severely intoxicated person requires medical backup; simply to let someone "sleep it off" unattended is to invite complications and even death. Stinson reports that prior to the commencement in 1967 of the alcoholism program in Rockford, Ill., there were an average of three alcoholic deaths a year in the local jail. As of early 1974, all 27 general hospitals in the area were admitting acute alcoholics, the police were cooperative and there had been no such deaths for 3 years. When the center opened, only 13 percent of its admissions had been detoxified under medical auspices; by 1974, the figure had risen to 94 percent.[9] The moral is obvious: while the principal task of a center is to give long-term treatment, a great deal of missionary work may have to be done to insure that the patient arrives there in good enough condition to make that most important part of his treatment possible.

Long-term treatment in the past has been severely crippled by several professional attitudes. The professional gives the patient his pet prescription, whatever it may be, and tells him to go and drink no more. The patient "falls off the wagon." The therapist blames the patient, not his own treatment, thereby "proving" that "alcoholics can't be helped" and reinforcing his own reluctance to treat them.

Alcoholism is a *chronic* disease, in this respect resembling diabetes or arthritis. To expect an alcoholic person never to relapse is about as sensible as to expect that a diabetic will never go out of control or that an arthritic never have a flareup.

In treating such disorders, the realistic physician understands full well that the best he can hope for in most cases is two steps forward, one step back. Perhaps the best analogy is that of rehabilitative medicine. The athlete who has been severely injured in an accident may never play football again, but if he can be taught, albeit slowly and painfully, to walk, use his hands, and again become a productive member of society, is this not something of which both he and his physician may be proud? Similarly, there are many hallmarks of "success" in the treatment of alcoholic people besides total abstinence. If, for example, a patient has been under threat of job dismissal, if his work performance is improved enough to remove or ameliorate that threat, if he then goes on a Saturday night binge, but is still able to show up sober on Monday morning, has he not been helped, and importantly so? Yet many physicians who would be pleased with a comparable degree of progress in a diabetic, condemn the alcoholic individual in such cases.

Of course, we want to do still better, and we should try to do so. This is yet another reason why it cannot be emphasized too strongly that treatment must be tailored to the needs of the individual patient. If one form of therapy does not work, try another, but above all do not expect that your patient will never regress. Alcoholic people are no more angels than the rest of us are.

There is one more vital element to successful treatment. The therapist must at all costs avoid a judgmental, moralistic attitude. The alcoholic person mortally fears rejection, yet invites it as evidence of his own unworthiness. He was "bad" and drank to assuage his guilt; now he has done an additional "bad thing" and is even guiltier; he faces his mentor like a cowering child, expecting to be punished, even provoking punishment ("Go ahead and hit me."). The patient may also react with belligerence and anger. It may sometimes be difficult for the therapist not to respond to the patient's anger by showing his own, but that must at all costs be avoided. However, calling the patient's attention to the effect his behavior has on others can be helpful in creating a new sense of self-awareness.

In truth, what both therapist and patient need to understand is that the very fact of the client's return to therapy is a victory for both of them. A major battle has been won, even though the war continues.

Destructive behavior often goes further than the verbal expression of anger. It may take the form of violence against the patient himself or others. Hertzman and Bendit suggest that alcoholic violence may follow an age-related pattern. In the younger years, this violence often is directed toward others—fights, barroom brawls, sometimes homicide—but, in later years, will more often result in suicide. In middle age, "accidental" deaths, such as traffic accidents, reach a peak.[19] Murphy and Robins found that alcoholic suicides very often occur within a year of a personal loss, e.g., death, separation, divorce. Even more importantly, in a study of 31 alcoholic suicides, they found that two-thirds of the suicides occurred within 6 weeks after the loss.[20] The implications for prevention are obvious. When losses occur or are anticipated, additional support must be offered to the patient. This should be continued for at least 6 weeks, and, if appropriate, the patient should be hospitalized.

We have talked much about the attitude of the therapist because we believe it to be the most important single factor in his success. It must be warm, helpful, supportive. Even a passive attitude on the part of the therapist, as distinct from a negative one, may be seen by the patient as rejection. On the other side of the coin, certain alcoholic patients show a passive resistance and dependence. The therapist must be sufficiently active to make the patient aware of this trait and to encourage him to work at his rehabilitation.

However, while it is essential that the patient have someone to whom he can relate for warmth and support, someone who is always there, person-to-person therapy alone has a dishearteningly low rate of success. We have pointed to some of the supporting elements that may be helpful, but there are also others.

Aversion therapy.   This is based on the theory that the patient is more likely to avoid alcohol if drinking has unpleasant associations. He is given emetine or apomorphine with alcohol, which produces nausea and vomiting. This form of conditioning seems to work best in patients who are in the higher socioeconomic groups and who have a sustained relationship with the therapist.

Disulfiram.   The patient who takes disulfiram (Antabuse) knows that if he later drinks even a small amount of alcohol, he will become violently, even dangerously, ill. Disulfiram is no longer regarded as the cure-all that enthusiasts once hoped it would become, but it is a useful crutch for many patients, who find it a substitute for "will power" while more deep-seated remedies are being sought.

Tranquilizers and other drugs.   A special word is in order about the use of minor tranquilizers such as chlordiazepoxide (Librium) and the alcoholic patient. These drugs have been widely prescribed in the hope that they will decrease the patient's anxiety and therefore his drinking. However, in too many instances, the drugs have been misused. Some patients develop an addiction to the drug that substitutes for the drug alcohol; others become addicted to the drug and continue drinking, adding one addiction to another. Such double addiction is complicated by the potentiating effects of the two drugs, which are both central nervous system depressants. There is recent evidence that antidepressants and major tranquilizers may be effective in treating the alcoholic patient.[21-24] With all tranquilizers, however, the prescribing physician should keep firmly in mind their synergistic effect with alcohol. Both he and the patient need to be sharply aware of the dangers involved.

One study has indicated that lithium carbonate, which is used in treatment and prophylaxis of the manic and hypomanic phases of manic-depressive illnesses, may be effective in preventing severe drinking bouts in patients who continue to drink.[25]

Drugs of any kind should never be used as a way of getting rid of an alcoholic patient. No matter how effective a particular chemical proves to be, recovery is still largely dependent on a good relationship between the patient and the therapist.

Group therapy.   Group therapy has become popular in recent years. Pioneered in its essential form by Alcoholics Anonymous (without guidance from the medical profession, be it noted), it has the advantage of economy, and it also appears to be more successful than individual treatment alone for many patients who can respond to the group's social interaction and are helped by seeing themselves through the eyes of other patients and by learning to see their relationships to others more clearly. For some patients, other techniques are also claimed to be helpful, among them transactional analysis, gestalt therapy, psychodrama, and transcendental meditation. The basic fact is that *any* technique must be fitted into an overall program tailored to the individual patient.

Alcoholics Anonymous.   AA is of benefit to perhaps more patients than any other single mode of assistance. This loosely organized fellowship has helped hundreds of thousands of alcoholic people to maintain sobriety. However, AA can only help those patients who accept its evangelistic approach or those who are ready to admit that they have ''hit bottom.''

The family.   Often, the alcoholic patient's family needs help as much as he does. The long-suffering wife who ''wants nothing more than her husband's recovery'' may actually ''need'' his alcoholism to fulfill a neurotic need of her own. It has been observed that sometimes when the alcoholic member of a family shows signs of improvement, his spouse begins to develop serious problems of her own.[26] Many therapists now routinely see the wife and often the children and other close relatives. They are brought together to examine their own roles in the problem and to make any necessary changes in their lives. An advantage of family therapy is not only that changes can be made to help prevent further drinking by the adult, or a family breakup, but it may also help to prevent alcoholism from developing in the patient's children.

Society.   Speck has focused on marshaling support for clients and their families from the wide range of people with whom they have close contact.[27] Such a network approach could enlist all the significant people in the patient's life, ranging from co-workers and neighbors to the bartender in his favorite saloon, to help the patient. This approach has only had limited application thus far.

FOLLOW-UP AND EVALUATION

Follow-up of alcoholic clients after the immediate crisis has passed is essential, not only so that success may be evaluated, but so that reinforcement may be offered as necessary. The question to be answered is, does the patient continue to function passably, and, if he senses danger, does he freely return for further help? Fortunately, the alcoholic population is a relatively stable one geographically, so long-term contact can be maintained with a large percentage of patients. Health maintenance organizations, for example, are in an especially advantageous position for follow-up; as the patient repeatedly returns to satisfy his other health-care needs, it is a simple matter to check on the state of his alcoholism.

Much of the follow-up work can be done advantageously and economically by paraprofessionals, so long as the professionals are on call if their services should be required. What is badly needed is financial support for followup by third-party payers. For a long while, they almost universally excluded alcoholism altogether from coverage; now some, although unfortunately too few, support acute care and a limited amount of therapy. It is tragic if a patient drops out of therapy or is not followed up for lack of money, and every effort should be made to prevent that.

No program can reach its full potential unless it is continually evaluated and steady improvement made. While it may be difficult or impossible to quantify the improvement in individual patients in precise percentages or neatly drawn graphs, it is not hard to be sure that someone has improved if he once could not hold a job and is now fruitfully employed. Measurements of self-esteem and self-image are used.* A strong subjective element is inevitable in anyone's assessment of patient improvement, but it can be balanced out at least to some extent by peer judgments. Perhaps even more importantly, the subjective views of the patients should be sought and weighed in with those of the staff.

One simple and useful criterion of success or failure is the number of dropouts from treatment. A high dropout rate means that someone, somewhere, in the organization is "turning off" substantial numbers of patients. It may be anyone from a cold therapist to a snippy receptionist, but it should not take much detective work to find the source of the trouble. Again, ask the patients!

Whatever methods of evaluation are used, there are really only two fundamental questions: are you helping as many people as possible as much as possible? If not, how can you do better?

ACKNOWLEDGMENTS

We gratefully acknowledge the assistance of Ann Noll, Jay Nelson Tuck, and Lynne Tuck, as well as the forebearance of the editor, in the preparation of this manuscript.

REFERENCES

1. NIAAA: Alcohol and alcoholism: problems, programs and progress. 1972, DHEW Publication No. (HSM) 72–9127. Washington, D.C., U.S. Govt. Printing Office, 1972.

2. Cahalan D: Problem Drinkers. San Francisco, Jossey-Bass, 1970

3. Cahalan D, Cisin IH, Crossly HM: American Drinking Practices: A National Survey of Drinking Behavior and Attitudes. New Haven, College and Univ Pr, 1969

4. Cahalan D, Room R: Problem drinking among American men. Monographs of the Rutgers Center of Alcohol Studies, No. 7.

*For example, in the Alcoholic Treatment Center Monitoring System of the NIAAA.

New Brunswick, N.J., 1972

5. Public awareness of an NIAAA advertising campaign and public attitudes toward drinking and alcohol abuse. Prepared for the National Instite on Alcohol and Alcoholism by Louis Harris & Associates, Inc., New York, 1972

6. World Health Organization, Quoted in Chafetz ME: Addictions. III. Alcoholism, in Freedman AM, Kaplan HI (eds): Comprehensive Textbook of Psychiatry, Baltimore, Williams & Wilkins, 1967, p 1011

7. Chafetz ME, Demone HW Jr.: Alcoholism & Society. New York, Oxford Univ Pr, 1962

8. Chafetz MD, Hill MJ: The alcoholic in society, in Grunebaum HU (ed): The Practice of Community Mental Health. New York, Little, Brown, 1970

9. Stinson D: Personal communication, Jan. 1974. Alcoholism Treatment Program, H. Douglas Singer Zone Center, Rockford, Ill.

10. Blane HT, Overton WF, Chafetz ME: Social factors in the diagnosis of alcoholism. 1. Characteristics of the patient. Q J Stud Alc 24:640–663, 1963

11. Criteria Committee, National Council on Alcoholism: Criteria for the diagnosis of alcoholism. Am J Psychiatry 129:2, 1972

12. NIAAA: From program to person: towards a national policy on alcoholism services. (in press)

13. Amark C: A study in alcoholism: Clinical, social-psychiatric and genetic investigations. Acta Psychiatr Neurol Scand suppl 70, 1951

14. Goodwin DW, Schulsinger F, Hermansen L, et al: Alcohol problems in adoptees raised apart from alcoholic biological parents. Arch Gen Psychiatry 28:238–243, 1973

15. Rose A, Burks B: Adult adjustment of foster children of alcoholic and psychotic parentage and the influence of the foster home. Memoirs of the Section on Alcohol Studies, New Haven, Yale University No. 3, Q J Stud Alc, 1945

16. Schuckit M, Goodwin DW, Winokur G: A study of alcoholism references in half siblings. Am J Psychiatry 128:1132–1136, 1972

17. Fenna D, Mix L, Schaefer O, et al: Ethanol metabolism in various racial groups. Can Med Assoc J 105, 472–475, 1971

18. Wolff PH: Ethnic differences in alcohol sensitivity. Science 175:449–450, 1972

19. Hertzmann M, Bendit EA: Alcoholism and destructive behavior, in Roberts A (ed): Self-Destructive Behavior, Springfield, Ill., Charles C Thomas (in press)

20. Murphy GE, Robins E: Social factors in suicide. JAMA 199:5, 1967

21. Butterworth AT: Depression associated with alcohol withdrawal; imipramine therapy compared with placebo. Q J Stud Alc 32:343–348, 1971

22. Butterworth AT, Watts RD: Treatment of hospitalized alcoholics with doxepin and diazepam; a controlled study. Q J Stud Alc 32:78–81, 1971

23. Overall JE, Brown D, Williams JD, et al: Drug treatment of anxiety and depression in detoxified alcoholic patients. Arch Gen Psychiatry 29:218–221, 1973

24. Hollister, LE, et al: Acetophenazine and diazepam in anxious depressions. Arch Gen Psychiatry 24:273–278, 1971

25. Kline NS: Evaluation of lithium therapy in chronic alcoholism. Paper presented before Third Annual Alcoholism Conference, NIAAA, 1973

26. Chafetz ME: Clinical syndromes of liquor drinkers, in Popham RE (ed): Alcohol & Alcoholism. Canada, Univ of Toronto Pr, 1970

27. Speck RV, Rueveni U: Network Therapy, Family Process. New York, Basic Books, 1970

PART III

Beyond the Community Mental Health Center

Robert L. Leopold, M.D.

9

Toward Health Maintenance Organization

THE COMMUNITY MENTAL HEALTH CENTER: A LOOK BACKWARD

The community mental health center (CMHC) at its inception gave promise of delivering much to many. As it has developed, it has indeed given much, but only to a relatively few, and at a disproportionately high cost. Despite some real accomplishments in the face of monumental difficulties—as documented so well in other chapters—many early hopes and expectations remain unfulfilled. Examples are such fundamental aims of the CMHC philosophy as a blanketing of the United States with several thousand centers, a massive program of primary prevention services, and a network of dependable and consistent continuity of care. Clearly the attainment through the CMHC of the goal of comprehensive, one-class coverage in the prevention and treatment of mental illness is a far more complex and expensive undertaking than was postulated at the CMHC's conception.

The current functioning of CMHCs must be viewed in the context of the expense of such centers, as well as in terms of their effectiveness and productivity. Only by critically examining the present status of the centers can one look toward the future place of the delivery of mental health services in the broad area of health care and welfare delivery systems.

Funding Problems

From the viewpoint of expense alone, there can be little doubt that the CMHC is at a critical point in its development. Current CMHC legislation expires on June 30, 1974, and the prospects for renewal are uncertain. Continuation

The help of Dorothy S. Kuhn, B.A., in compiling the data presented here is gratefully acknowledged.

grants for programs already funded will go on until their authorization periods end. For example, a program in the first year of the staffing grant legislation (1965) lost support at the end of June, 1973. Thus, grants currently in existence expire annually until the end of fiscal 1981. In addition, CMHCs are eligible to apply for federal support under a number of other mental health programs. They expire at different times, with some having run out in June, 1973.

The fate of the CMHC funding legislation remains questionable. If federal support is withdrawn or reduced significantly, as may well be the case, it appears highly improbable that state and local governments will make up the difference in funding. Thus, if CMHCs wish to expand, and if new ones are to be developed, there will be an increased need for funds at the same time that current funds are being withdrawn.

At best, CMHCs will be able to operate in relatively few geographical areas. Financing, if available at all, will flow mainly through Title XVIII and Title XIX of the Social Security Act, and through various other social service streams, and in effect will be allocated chiefly to serve the elderly, the impoverished, and the unemployable. In other words, funding will have to come from multiple sources, which will include the diminishing income from grants, payments from third parties, and consultation contracts from government and nongovernment sources. Each source is likely to earmark its funds for a specific kind of activity. Funding agencies are usually (and understandably) zealous in protecting their own terrains, and so demand substantial accountability. Logically, then, programs will be developed in relation to existing funding sources, often to the detriment of an overall, well-planned program base.

In contrast, the general health care system is looking forward to single-payment funding for all personal health care services. The mechanism may be third-party insurance, national health insurance, direct government subsidy, fee for service, or a combination of these. Whatever the mechanism, the point at issue is that a single payment for each person covered, derived from funds specifically intended for personal health care, is expected to cover all agreed-upon services. Thus the allocation of resources may rest on a far more rational base than will be the case with the CMHC system.

The CMHC, left to the mercy of the multiple mandates emanating from various supporting systems, will be faced with increasingly difficult choices.[1,2] Under stringent accountability regulations, service providers tend to resort to more and more subterfuge and rationalization, action which is hardly conducive to their own mental health. In the nature of things, the holders of the purse strings are likely to win the escalating struggle to protect their own terrains. The consumer ultimately is the loser: At best, he is offered unlinked and incoherent services responding to needs that may not necessarily include his own; at worst, no relevant services are available.

Despite the mammoth financial difficulties indicated here, some CMHCs will probably manage to maintain themselves in one way or another for a few years. Less likely is the possibility that new CMHCs will be established in numbers bearing any realistic relation to need. On the contrary, as Schwartz suggests,[3] existing CMHCs are likely to be forced to serve larger and larger populations, with consequently less and less individualized care. The CMHC system, he comments, before long will begin to look curiously like the old state hospital system. There is no need here to enlarge on that unhappy but quite realistic projection. What should be emphasized, rather, is that the future, financially speaking, seems to hold little long-term promise for the CMHC system as a separate social institution charged with the implementation of the community mental health approach.

The rapidly escalating costs of mental health programs are well known. One small example will suffice: In Pennsylvania, the state mental health/mental retardation budget has increased from $18 million in the fiscal year 1968–1969 to over $61 million in the fiscal year 1972–1973. Significantly, the $61 million represents $12 million less than the governor requested of the legislature. These figures do not include the 10 percent matching funds legislatively obligated as county contributions to mental health/mental retardation services. The magnitude of increase represents the anticipated increases in federal and local budgets for the developing mental health programs. It is clear that there is no popular mandate to fund programs at this magnitude, even if the monies were potentially available.

In short, I believe that adequate funding mechanisms for perpetuating the community mental health center as it currently exists—i.e., as a separate system for implementing the community mental health approach—are not now present and will not exist in the foreseeable future. The problem confronting us in 1974 is not survival as a separate system, but rather survival of the positive accomplishments of the CMHC in the sense of furthering the community mental health approach. Instead of hoping vainly that money to continue the CMHCs will somehow materialize, it seems more useful to look beyond the centers toward a future for the community mental health approach in which the weaknesses of the centers can be remedied and their strengths perpetuated.

Evaluation of the Program

Predicting the future is a hazardous undertaking. Evaluation of the assets of the community mental health approach is necessarily subjective, and indeed problems of evaluation of center activities have been almost as serious as the problems of financing the centers. Thus, we are without adequate objective evaluative guidelines as we attempt to justify that which we would feel to be useful in the CMHC approach. No one has as yet defined either mental health or mental illness in terms specific enough to measure accurately the overall effects on any population of so massive a treatment and prevention program as that attempted by the CMHC. Thus, the author must use criteria that are at best subjective, impressionistic, colored by observer bias, and utterly without consensual validation.

Under the circumstances, any statement he may make is likely to lean heavily on personal experience. This chapter is indeed a frankly personal statement based on the following experience: many years in private practice, with concomitant consultant work in developing clinical and preventive mental health services for the American Friends Service Committee and—more recently—the Peace Corps; 5 years, after leaving private practice, as director of the West Philadelphia Community Mental Health Consortium (a CMHC); and, after resigning that post, as chairman of the department of community medicine of a university medical school. The present position, offering a window on the wider world of general health care delivery, has strengthened a personal conviction held since earliest CMHC experience: If the community mental health approach is to survive as a viable instrument for delivering mental health care commensurate with the state of our knowledge, it must join forces with the health care system.

STRENGTH, WEAKNESS, AND DIFFUSION OF EFFORT

Like many another system devised to improve the human condition, the CMHC derives many of its weaknesses from its strengths. Surely no one will deny that a fundamental strength rests in its view of the individual and his problems, a view that takes into account both the internal and external forces that contribute to his existence and includes, hopefully, much that is relevant in the thinking of medicine as well as of all other disciplines that concern themselves with human well-being. Nevertheless, despite its undeniable worth, the CMHCs holistic view has been subjected to other forces in such a way as to produce a striking weakness: diffusion of effort. Indeed, in this author's view, the most trying problems the CMHCs have had to face, and particularly those in urban areas, can be subsumed under that single rubric.

One such force is the catchment area concept. The division of the United States into catchment areas for CMHC purposes was proposed as a means of focusing mental health effort into discrete, geographically defined areas of responsibility. If one recalls that one of the main objectives of the CMHC legislation was the emptying of state hospitals and the return of patients to their former communities, the concept, by making the previous or current place of residence a salient planning feature, was sound. One must also recall that state hospital patients tend to come largely from socially and economically deprived population segments. Geographically defined catchment areas therefore served in general to divide the country into affluent and impoverished regions. To make matters worse, catchment area boundaries frequently took little account of other functional boundaries, such as those for police districts, political subunits, educational districts, and general health planning units, so that in many catchment areas there is a significant shortage of human service agencies other than the CMHC. At the same time, since most states use catchment area boundaries only for mental health funding, they bear little relationship to other health and welfare funding units. In short, in the many catchment areas characterized by extreme social and economic deprivation and a shortage of relevant ameliorative agencies, social needs were almost immediately seen by those living in the area as having a far more urgent priority than mental health needs.

One cannot, of course, banish poverty by districting a system in one way rather than in another. But the catchment area concept has unquestionably placed a disproportionate share of poverty's burden on those CMHCs that could afford it least. In fact, in a corrective effort, additional federal monies were made available in the late 1960s to catchment areas that met certain poverty criteria. But it is doubtful whether any amount of mental health money could reasonably have been expected to solve problems of the extent and magnitude found in these areas.

The major question here, however, is whether a mental health agency should be given the responsibility for attempting to solve these social problems. At this point, it becomes necessary to look at another force that has helped to create diffusion of effort out of the holistic view. For want of a better term, and without disrespect, one might call this force the "prevention syndrome." To the mental health professions, "prevention" has a mystical aura. For many reasons that need not be reviewed here, during several decades immediately preceding and the one following the inauguration of the CMHC, the aura attached itself to the tempting possibilities for prevention inherent in interventions in the social environment. Indeed, the mental health professions (as well as related behavioral science disciplines) allowed themselves to be overwhelmed by the aura to the extent of believing, with undoubted sincerity, that social reform and the prevention of mental illness are almost synonymous. No one questions the desirability of prevention, but unfortunately, no one knows, in the context of mental illness, what it really means, how to do it, or how to measure it. The multiple causes of mental illness make the evaluation of single interventions in the environment impossible. Even where more data are available, as in certain family situations, the range of variables makes certainty unlikely. Yet the attractiveness of prevention through social action has seduced the CMHC into periods of frenetic activity, in which doing something is equated with doing something useful. The continuing absence of clear guidelines from the National Institute of Mental Health about the CMHC's proper role in this sphere has not helped.

I do not wish to deny the association, now generally recognized, between mental illness and social need, but simply to point out my conviction that the CMHC has little or no expertise at its disposal that it might usefully apply to direct action in the vast sphere of urban problems. More specifically, such concerns as delinquency, housing, sanitation, minimum family income, job discrimination, and other socioeconomic issues are not productive areas in which the CMHC should expend its funds and energies. Too often, clinical services and consultation and education services that might serve the consumer's needs with more immediacy and pertinence than social reform have been abrogated in favor of poorly conceived and unevaluated social action programs which, however desirable, should be undertaken by agencies specifically designed to do so. Despite these considerations, whether some CMHCs have made significant progress in the sphere of social action is impossible to measure on any useful scale. It can only be reemphasized that expenditures of time and effort in this direction have occurred at the expense of more direct services.

Perhaps more important, diffusion of effort has caused many persons in the CMHC's consumer community to evaluate the function of the CMHC not on the grounds of its appropriate mission, but on the basis of an individual's own feeling of what a CMHC should be doing in the field of social action. For example, to someone concerned primarily with housing, the fact that a CMHC has made little impact on improving the housing situation in its catchment area is convincing evidence of the failure of that CMHC, regardless of how well it may be treating ill people or detecting illness in its early stages. Since social problems of the magnitude confronting some CMHCs have proved insoluble despite the efforts of many agencies over many years, the CMHC, when judged on such grounds, is obviously in a no-win situation.

Moreover, as the CMHC has moved into the social action sphere, it has become increasingly the object of political maneuvering and confrontation. Its agenda is thus frequently perverted by the agenda of interest groups who are competing against each other for its attention, and the center finds itself then struggling not only with socioeconomic problems beyond its competence, but also with sociopolitical issues about which it likewise has little or no knowledge and over which it cannot possibly have any control. This is not to repeat what has been said in previous paragraphs, but to suggest the ever-spiraling nature of diffusion of effort. In other words, the more the CMHC moves into the social action field, the more it is pressured politically into additional efforts. Vitiation of attempts to deliver direct mental health services spirals upward, while the CMHC diverts more and more of its resources to other purposes. It tends to fail in its primary mandate because it is overinvolved in areas where it has little chance to accomplish anything.

Community involvement, a significant and valued component of the CMHC approach, has, unfortunately, also been responsible for much diffusion of effort. The term "community involvement" is used to connote consumer participation in the decision-making processes, where mental health services, intended for his benefit, are planned and delivered. I shall not attempt to argue the merits of the various degrees of community involvement. My purpose here is simply to point out that the response by the CMHC to the rising demand for community involvement has been the expenditure of large amounts of resources. The fact that the legislative and regulatory guidelines are generally vague has compounded the problem.

There can be no question that the consumer not only should, but must, participate in defining, planning, and delivering services intended for his benefit. There are differences of opinion in respect mainly to the degree of participation; these in turn have generated some differences in terminology. Thus Bolman,[4] for example, in a thoughtful review, prefers the term "community control," whereas I prefer "community involvement." Either term suggests the amount of time and effort which has been necessary to integrate a new government structure into a rudimentary care system. One of the most significant aspects of the community mental health approach has been the opportunity it has afforded to include the community in the decisions of what had previously been the self-arrogated privilege of the provider to define need according to his own lights and then to respond idiosyncratically to the need as the professional sees it. Nevertheless, the opportunity to effect significant changes by maximizing community involvement in a way which may well be unique for a service delivery system has also served to draw the attention of the system away from its primary goals. The consumer's rising interest is particularly hard to resist when it is encountered in the face-to-face situations that must ensue when the consumer is invited to enter the planning and decision-making process. There it works rapidly to induce the provider to expand his definitions of mental health, and therefore his range of activities, until his activities become practically coterminal with that of the consumer. The result is all too often chaos, with the inevitable breakdown of an orderly delivery system.[5]

CONSULTATION AND EDUCATION

Consultation and education to community agencies and professional personnel constitute another area that can scarcely be discussed without reference to diffusion of effort. Here commitment (perhaps overcommitment) to the holistic view, the prevention syndrome, and inadequate legislative and regulatory guidelines has produced a monumental range of interpretations and misinterpretations of the fifth of the five essential services mandated by the initial Community Mental Health Center Act. Without wishing to add to the debate, I feel obliged to state here my own view that consultation and education should be strictly clinical adjunctives. In this view, consultation means *mental health* consultation as Caplan[6] conceives it: A means of spreading available professional expertise to promote maximal utilization of limited clinical resources. Education means a program of instruction for persons connected with mental-health-related agencies (e.g., teachers and parents in the school system; policemen and guards in a criminal justice system; youth leaders and parents in a church-based organization) who are not expected to render clinical care. Such a program will enable them to understand a few broad and elementary aspects of health and mental illness to the end that they will be able to recognize their manifestations and make appropriate referrals for treatment.

Both consultation and education, of course, have been extended to include activities far outside this limited view. Indeed, it is often difficult to see even what is perceived as education and what as consultation. Some activities loosely grouped under "consultation and education" apparently seek to make complete diagnosticians and clinicians out of everyone in the community; others aim to teach the poor how to seek correction for major socioeconomic problems. In the one case, there is no denying that a well-informed public can help with early identification of patients and bringing them to treatment; but even for consultees, as well as the general public, there is a point at which information is useless or even harmful. In the other case, certainly the poor and powerless might benefit from learning how to take social action, but mental health personnel are rarely qualified to teach in this context, even if such teaching were an appropriate activity for the CMHC.

A focal point of tension between providers and consumers has grown out of the consultation and education issue. The providers have tended to believe that such services are good, ipso facto, and many CMHCs have made strenuous and often successful attempts to allocate to them quite substantial resources. The consumer almost universally (and paradoxically, this is true even when the consumer community also looks to the CMHC for social action) has assigned consultation and education a lower priority than has the provider and has importuned for more direct services. It may be that consumer wisdom exceeds provider wisdom if one considers, for example, that direct clinical intervention in a single family may have a higher prevention payoff than many indirect services believed, without much foundation in fact, to affect the mental health of the community—such as any number of lectures to school and church groups.

Even within the limited view of the function of consultation and education held by this author, it must be emphasized that these services do act as case-finding mechanisms. This presents a spiraling problem of resource allocation. No one doubts the value of case finding, yet the more the CMHC offers consultation and education, the more it is likely to be pressured for additional clinical service which it may not have enough staff to provide. Nevertheless, if consultation and education are kept within the boundaries suggested here, at least resources will be conserved for dealing with increased clinical demands, rather than dissipated in activities that lie outside the mandate in the field of mental health.

In any case, many CMHCs have in fact developed consultation and education services that fulfill a useful clinical adjunctive purpose; and all, even by honoring this purpose in the breach, have helped many persons to define their views more precisely. The consultation and education concept, despite flaws in interpretation, must be counted among the strengths of the CMHCs that should be perpetuated no matter what direction the community mental health approach may take.

MENTAL RETARDATION PROGRAMS

Mental retardation is another problem that falls under the rubric of diffusion of effort, although it cannot be traced to quite the same roots as those previously discussed. Mental retardation was engrafted onto the CMHC system for political reasons that need not be reviewed here. Suffice it to say that the mental health system, in order to be funded, had to take on mental retardation. This is a curious anomaly, since those most active in the field regard mental retardation as primarily neither a psychiatric nor a medical question, but as an educational matter—one for professional teachers and others who are interested in educating all human beings to the limits of their capacities. Certainly the mentally retarded person who is also psychiatrically ill is a legitimate concern of the CMHC. But it is difficult to see why, rationally, the CMHC should be expected to develop programs specifically designed for the whole range of retardation needs, including education, rehabilitation, day care, residence, and transportation. Mental health professionals are rarely equipped to deal adequately with these needs. When the CMHC, under political and financial pressure, attempts to respond to them, it diverts resources that should be available for mental health care for all persons, regardless of their level of mental development. And once more, when the CMHC fails to respond satisfactorily in a sphere where it has little or no competence, it is judged on the basis of that failure, regardless of what it may have achieved in treatment of the mentally ill.

At present, there seems to be no clear-cut resolution of this problem in sight, regardless of what future lies "beyond the CMHC" for the community mental health approach. Certainly the medically ill retarded person is a legitimate concern of the general health care system, yet no more than the CMHC can that system be expected rationally to provide a full range of services for the retarded. Perhaps the most that can be said within the charge of this chapter is that those who have been, or will be, unjustly burdened with this responsibility will have to demand that state and local education departments gradually take over existing programs and develop future services. Certainly this responsibility must include tapping whatever funding resources are available from federal agencies.

SUMMARY

At this point, I should like to summarize briefly what I see as the essential meaning to be extracted from the foregoing inventory. The CMHC, in being forced to function as an all-purpose social welfare agency, has failed on two counts: (1) as an all-purpose social welfare agency, because it lacks the necessary knowledge and resources; (2) as a clinical agency, because it has diverted to the functions of an all-purpose social welfare agency too many of the limited resources it has had for clinical work. Not all CMHCs have tried to function as all-purpose social welfare agencies. I believe one can safely say that more have than not, simply because CMHCs are likely most often to be established in areas where there is the greatest need for both mental health and social welfare resources. By and large, the CMHC's failure seems to be built into the system—not so much the system as initially conceptualized, but the system as it has evolved from a complicated mixture of interpretations of the CMHC's goals and functions contributed by both providers and users. Whatever the process that has produced the mixture, the CMHC is now perceived by substantial numbers of people as an all-purpose social welfare agency rather than a clinical agency. In other words, the CMHC has tended to move increasingly into the welfare system and out of the health care system. I believe this movement is a more significant and a more basic loss for the community mental health approach than the failure of the CMHC itself.

That approach evolved at least in large part from an urgent need to take the mentally ill out of the welfare system. For a variety of financial and medical reasons, the state hospital, where so many of the mentally ill were "treated" for so many years in the United States, was and continues to be a welfare institution. As such, it perpetuated a two-class care system (one for the affluent, one for the nonaffluent) without any substantial interruption until well after World War II. Whatever else was hoped for the community mental health approach, it was envisioned as a passport to one-class care. The CMHC, by moving the community mental health approach into the welfare system, seems destined to destroy the dream. In a mixed economy, it seems to me impossible to foresee any other ultimate outcome for this movement but two-class care: superior care for the affluent, inferior care for the nonaffluent.

There seems no way to escape the conclusion that the CMHC's weaknesses and its consequent failures are rooted in its movement into the welfare system.

There would then seem to be only one logical answer if the community mental health approach is to survive the CMHC in such a way as to ameliorate its weaknesses and perpetuate its strengths. That answer is to take the approach out of the welfare system. I have already stated where I am convinced it should be taken: into the general health care system. Hopefully, it will take into the general health care system its many strengths in the treatment of the mentally ill, in the new and innovative uses of manpower, some of the refinements developed in the education and consultation process, its ease of access to treatment, and particularly its emphasis on the continuity of care.

MERGER OF MENTAL AND GENERAL HEALTH CARE:
A LOOK FORWARD

It is the thesis of this chapter that the community mental health approach cannot stand alone and be perpetuated indefinitely as a CMHC. The approach developed by the community mental health programs further appears to defeat its own purpose as part of the welfare system. Accordingly, it seems clear that, for the community mental health approach to continue to exert an influence on the health care system, it must in fact become part of the general health care system. The experience and knowledge gained during the past decade can be translated in meaningful terms for the developing health care system. If this does not occur, it seems likely that the approach will be lost along with the center. Put another way, and more crassly: Many readers may disagree with the thought that the mental health system must join the general health care delivery system. Unless, however, another home can be found, the health care system is the only game in town for those who want to be part of the community mental health action. Some practitioners may prefer a retreat to private practice, while others may prefer to turn their energies to the welfare field. To this author, however, the gradual, planned, and purposeful merger into the health care system is the opportunity most likely to afford furtherance of the community mental health approach.

It is no secret that the health care system is moving slowly and unevenly from what has been characterized as a cottage industry to one in which a systematic approach to the problem of care is being organized. Such an approach makes mandatory the use of a variety of kinds of manpower with specialized skills, and renders somewhat obsolete the master craftsman and his apprentices (for which one can read "the medical chief and his Indians"). No attempt will be made here to deal comprehensively with the evolving health care system. For such information, the reader is referred to works by Freidson[7] and Freeman et al.[8]

From the mental health standpoint, the salient factor is that the health care system is a *developing* one. It is still in a considerable state of flux, and indeed, one might add, in crisis. Since systems in crisis, like patients in crisis, are most amenable to intervention during acute periods of stress, the health care system is at an appropriate point for mental health consultation. By sharing with our colleagues many of the bitterly learned lessons of the past decade, we can enable a stronger delivery system to be established. Without attempting to be inclusive, the remainder of this chapter attempts to summarize the trends relevant to these times.

Changes in Medical Practice

The gradual disappearance of the individual medical practitioner, particularly from the inner city, is well known. There is a growing trend from solo to group practice, i.e., a movement from individual to team involvement in the care of patients. Comprehensive group practices are being developed in all parts of the country, in rural and urban settings, with family physicians, general internists, and pediatricians as core members of the group. As groups expand, their memberships may come to include gynecologists, obstetricians, general surgeons, radiologists, dentists, and others. Few groups, except the very largest, currently include psychiatrists. Other medical specialists are available as needed in the smaller comprehensive practices.

These groups are in the process of redefining the role of the physician in much the same way as the CMHC has been forced to redefine the role of the psychiatrist. However, quite unlike the mental health center in which the psychiatrist was pushed further and further away from his clinical base, the physician in a comprehensive group practice is able to deal increasingly with strictly medical affairs. Other members of the comprehensive team assume the nonmedical functions, ranging from administration to health education. This permits the economical employment of diverse skills, and at the same time permits the physician to deal in his own area of expert knowledge. Rather than diffusion of resources, this trend portends effective manpower utilization. In essence, the trend is toward appropriate use of medical and paramedical personnel in the health care area. Nonhealth activities remain the concern of more suitable institutions, since it is not economically feasible for the health system to become involved in areas outside its own field. The group practice maintains the responsibility for appropriate linkages to the entire human resources network and must devise means of monitoring and reinforcing these linkages. The problem-oriented medical record may facilitate this linkage.[9]

The organization into group practices facilitates the transfer of service emphasis from inpatient care to ambulatory center. In response to the pressures of escalating costs and consumer demands, the ambulatory care facility is increasingly becoming the center of the health care delivery system. This permits emphasis on earlier diagnosis and treatment, with less interruption of family continuity and employment function and with diminished costs. In the usual case, the group practice has community hospital facilities available to it, and its members follow the group's patients throughout their hospitalization. As the number of people covered by annual capitation increases so that the annual fee covers both outpatient and inpatient care, the ambulatory care facility and the community hospital become nodal points for the delivery system. Highly complex procedures can be expected increasingly to take place at the regional teaching center. However, the mechanisms for financial provision of these services remain unclear.

The reorganization of the forms of practice has been hastened by the increasing awareness of the cost of hospital care. As the new system emerges, one can expect that every effort will be made to limit the use of hospital beds to those patients who need treatment for their severe illnesses or who have highly specialized diagnostic needs, i.e., for patients who need secondary or tertiary care. The major emphasis will be on primary care, which can be defined as ambulatory care of ordinary illnesses given in an accessible, comprehensive manner within reasonable geographical proximity to the home or place of work. Those patients too ill for ambulatory care ideally will be seen in secondary care hospital facilities, and only those patients whose needs require elaborate and sophisticated technology will be transferred to tertiary care facilities. Within the group practice model, every effort is being made to guarantee the individual physician and patient contact throughout at least the entire primary and secondary care experience.[10]

Consumer Involvement

Individuals have demands for special kinds of services, which they see themselves as requiring when ill. At the same time, the health care professional perceives certain large requirements of the health care system in general and has tended to give these needs higher priority. The needs and demands of the individual patient and of the professional provider are often not congruent, and in the past the provider's perception, and his subsequent allocation of resources, has prevailed. Since the patient has not been able to enter a truly competitive market, he has, to this point, been forced to accept those services which the provider makes available to him. The provider of services has been the major determiner of what services will be offered and to whom. For example, the establishment of a cobalt machine or a renal dialysis unit may have a higher priority than the establishment of an accessible neighborhood health center. Thus, the provider has been the major determiner of how scarce monetary resources, both public and private, will be allocated. Insufficient attention has been paid to the expectations of individual patients for services.

As Boulding points out: "The activity originates from the profession rather than from the client, from the supplier rather than the demander. In its extreme form, it takes on the flavor of 'what you need is what I as your professional advisor have to give you. What you want is irrelevant.' "[11]

With "provider knows best" as the prevailing attitude, it is small wonder that the entire health and mental health care systems are being forced to respond to the demands of the consumer. Supported by federal guidelines, particularly in the area of services to impoverished persons, the consumer has seized increasing control of health care facilities. Not only was "maximum feasible participation" virtually mandated for projects funded by the Office of Economic Opportunity, including health projects, but also experimental funding was made available directly to local groups which received support and resources based on their assessment of local need.

While the impact of such representation has been questionable in terms of the actual acquiring of control, there can be little doubt that there is increased awareness on the part of the professional about the demands of those he serves.[12]

Methods of Compensation

The reader is, of course, familiar with current methods of compensation in the health care field. Care is paid for overwhelmingly on a fee-for-service basis for those able to pay. While a significant majority of individuals carry some form of third-party health insurance, the majority of these plans pay maximally the total benefits for inpatient care. Virtually no fee-for-service third-party arrangements pay for comprehensive costs. As could be expected, a dual-track system has evolved in which those who are employed or otherwise have means pay either directly for services or purchase insurance directly or as a result of labor contract benefits. Those not covered in this way, the medically indigent, under 65, have available only the modest benefits paid directly to providers by the state and local governments. Since these benefits generally pay fees far below the ordinary fees, such patients are forced into crowded and often undignified public facilities where services are characterized by impersonality, long waits for treatment, and little continuity of care. A form of national health insurance is available for those over 65 years of age in the medicare arrangements, which make use of the usual vendor of medical services in the treatment of episodes of illness. The costs of medicare have become extremely high, and there has been a gradual rise in the copayment component.

Some 8 million people in the United States are covered by single-payment annual fees for comprehensive medical services operating under a variety of auspices, a mechanism usually known as capitation.[13] (Examples are Kaiser-Permanente groups, Puget Sound Group Health Association, and Health Insurance Plan of New York City.) While data are not complete, it appears that single capitation payments afford the opportunity for more accessible, continuous, and earlier service at less cost, since in these plans the emphasis is on ambulatory rather than on hospital care. It thus seems likely that the fee-for-service payment mechanism will be replaced over time by a single annual payment to a health care provider. The payment may be made either directly to a health service organization (such as a health maintenance organization or medical foundation), or to such an organization from a fiscal intermediary, which may be one of the Blue plans or another insurer. Moreover, it is quite possible that for some individuals, such as those who receive medical assistance monies (Title XIX), the government may pay the capitation fee to the provider.

It is to be stressed that the important consideration here is not the structure of any particular health maintenance organization, but the concept of a single annual payment for total personal health services. The burden thus is thrust on the provider to detect illness early in its course and to prevent serious disability and hospitalization, since the "profits" to the provider depend upon the ways in which he manages the annual premium. Put another way, if the provider overutilizes the budgeted hospital resources available for his patient, he bears the cost.

Single-Payment Financing

In the capitation plan already in existence, a variety of provisions are available for mental health care.[14] It has been demonstrated quite effectively that a yearly payment of $8 to $12 per person would be sufficient to offer comprehensive coverage for mental illness in a prepaid health insurance plan. This is a small fraction of the total cost of such a package, and yet would include not only substantial inpatient care, but also perhaps 15 outpatient visits a year with copayment above that, some days of partial hospitalization, and considerable drug benefits.

It is to be anticipated that a universal health insurance policy will serve to mitigate the current two-class system of health care. Annual capitation from whatever source will provide the consumer of services with a discrete and clearly delineated package of health and illness benefits. The component parts of the basic coverage will most likely be stipulated by law. These are expected to include ambulatory, diagnostic, and hospital services. A floor will be placed on benefits available to all insured persons, whether the insurance is on a private or government basis.

As with any insurance package, however, it will be possible for more affluent persons to purchase more comprehensive coverage. This additional coverage may be in the form of more extended services or may permit more luxurious accommodations. Nevertheless, the fact that the basic, required group of benefits is available to all persons would establish the foundation for a unitary care system. Indeed, Public Law 92-603 allows medicare to pay an annual capitation fee to a provider with the stipulation that no more than 50 percent of the group enrolled by the provider are medicare recipients. The financing mechanisms are still rudimentary and many options are open.

Even in its present somewhat chaotic state in terms of financing and in terms of organization, the health care system presents some strong advantages from the standpoint of the mental health system. First, it is not, to any significant extent, guilty of diffusion of effort. If anything, its critics feel that it defines its role in treating illness rather than maintaining health too narrowly. Second, its function and accordingly its legitimization are clear: The health care system is in the health care business.

Similarity of Problems

It is significant that some of the problems which beset the health care system are similar to those which confronted the mental health care system at the inception of CMHCs. A central problem in mental health care was the position and relative importance of the state hospitals, and indeed, one could write the history of the mental health legislation in terms of an attempt to solve the state hospital problem. For very different reasons, the health care system currently is structured around the tertiary care hospital, which is expensive, inaccessible, and to a significant degree casts its spell over the whole system. Decentralization of care from the tertiary hospital to secondary and primary ambulatory care facilities is as important in the health system as it was in the mental health system, but it is far less likely to be accompanied by the diffusion of effort which characterized mental health ambulatory operations. The mandate for the care of the ill is quite clear in the health care system. There is a lesser mandate for the maintenance of health, but no significant mandate for the incursion into all of society's problems. It would be extraordinarily difficult to pervert the current health care system into wider social action, in part because of the widespread recognition that persons prepared to give medical care have no discrete expert welfare technology—a recognition which is not accorded the mental health worker.

The health care system thus starts with a much more clearly defined clinical base, and the movement from tertiary to ambulatory care is accordingly more likely to remain clinically oriented. There continues to be a division in the ranks of health planners concerning the utilization of major resources in primary preventive care such as automated annual physical examinations and mass screening studies, since the value of these activities is still quite uncertain. Other planners feel there are sufficient data to justify major allocation of resources in these areas. It is to be noted, however, that there is minimal or no pressure on the health care system to deliver services beyond the scope of a rather narrowly defined health experience.

The CMHC has shown that where everyone is practicing prevention, few are left to treat the ill. This is particularly true when prevention is interpreted in the diffuse manner which has become customary for mental health centers. It seems reasonable to believe that the more directly preventive services are linked to the known causes of illness, the more productive these efforts will be and the more measurable.

Thus, as mental health services become incorporated under the rubric of the health care system, the diffusion of so-called preventive effort will be lessened, and the expansion of early recognition and early treatment of disease in the clinical model will be expedited.

Not only will the structure of the emerging health care system limit the diffusion of effort by the mental health worker, but also it should enhance his effectiveness. He, with other members of the team, will be involved in an effort on behalf of a defined population, and should serve a unique function by handling those human and emotional problems which are within his professional competence to treat and by facilitating linkage with other sources which have available skills which he and others in the health care system lack. The painfully learned concept of a human network resource need not be abandoned. Rather, the mental health profession should become the leader in developing interfaces between the health care system and other relevant systems.

The opportunity to accomplish the effective merger of the health, mental health, and social service systems may be offered more quickly than had been anticipated.* In January 1972, President Nixon, in his State of the Union message, expressed his concern to the nation regarding the delivery of social services, and suggested the need for state and local mechanisms to coordinate their efforts. He elaborated this concern in a special message, "Delivery of Social Services," on May 18, 1972. His message urged the passing of the Allied Services Act, which proposed to correct the situation whereby "a compassionate Government unwillingly created a bureaucratic jungle that baffles and short-changes many citizens in need." This proposed legislation is being pretested currently by 20 social service demonstration projects funded in part from the Social and Rehabilitation Services, the Health Services, and Mental Health Administration, the Office of Education, and the Office of Child Development. Thus, health and mental health services are being joined with social, educational, and developmental services to help overcome the fragmented care from which many people suffer. The Social and Rehabilitation Service Administration has major responsibility for these projects, serving as the lead agency for 17 of the 20.

A key provision of the Allied Services Act is a listing of the human services program which *must* be coordinated and those which *may* be coordinated. Thus, no fewer than three of the following services must be coordinated:

1. Child welfare services
2. Vocational rehabilitation services for older Americans
3. Certain aspects of the Juvenile Delinquency Prevention and Control Act
4. Medicaid
5. Certain services under the Community Mental Health Services Act
6. Certain developmental disability services
7. Adult education services

At the federal level, then, an effort which to some may seem premature is being attempted to gather health, mental health, and nonhealth services into one coherent service system. While these pilot projects are per se of considerable interest and importance, their real significance lies in what they portend for the future.

Community Involvement

The developing health care delivery system has the responsibility to read well the lessons learned over the last decade by the CMHC experience. During this time, many CMHCs have fallen between the Scylla of overinvolvement and the Charybdis of underinvolvement. There are few workers in the health care delivery field who do not recognize that community involvement is a necessary and permanent component of delivery systems. How well such community involvement serves the community depends, at least in part, on how certain the health provider is of

*The author is indebted to Dr. Stanley J. Brody, Associate Professor of Social Planning, Department of Community Medicine and Department of Psychiatry, University of Pennsylvania, for gathering the material which follows.

his own professional competence, and how great his determination is to stick to his professional last. Within his competence, there are a variety of methods of delivery and priorities of service, the choice of which may well be theprerogative of the consumer. For example, if a hospital has a finite amount of money to spend, should it spend funds to reequip the emergency ward or to add equipment for open-heart surgery? Assuming that the professional staff knows equally well how to make proper use of either kind of equipment, the determination to allocate the funds properly might well be a nonprofessional decision. However, this author believes that it is not proper for the community to decide which antibiotic to use for a specific infection. In his own experience as director of a mental health center whose board of directors had equal voting membership from the community and from member agencies, community representatives were eager to make the first kind of decision, often on the basis of a clearer perception of need than that of professionals, and loath to make the second kind of decision, which they had no difficulty in perceiving as a professional issue. The consumer members of the board were deeply concerned with the appearance of neighborhood clinics and with assurance of adequate staffing of these clinics; but they resented any attempt to persuade them to join in decisions regarding the kind of clinical treatment the staff should use in particular cases.

The CMHC, both as an institution and as an approach to the problem of health care delivery, has been a forerunner in bringing consumers in the ranks of determiners of service. Unfortunately, even now few formal guidelines are available, since what has been learned has been in the area of process rather than in the development of a set of rigid criteria. Reports of such process are available, [5,15-17] and perusal of these reports would give the reader a sense of the similarities and the differences involved. It is to be hoped that an attempt will be made to summarize these experiences for the use of the emerging health care system. It is certainly likely that the general health care delivery system will encounter the same problems with respect to community involvement as has the mental health care delivery system. As yet, no easy answers have emerged. It is clear that the professional in either field, in his urgent wish to do everything requested of him by the community, must guard against ending up doing nothing. Perhaps community involvement is regarded best as an educational process in which providers and users, as partners, learn from each other what is possible to accomplish, what is not possible to accomplish, and what can be effected. Certainly some CMHCs have set such a process in motion. Whatever the fate of the CMHC, its leaders—no matter how badly they have been battered by the experience of setting the process in motion—can take comfort in the fact that community involvement is now a meaningful reality in at least one part of the health care system.

Complementarity of the Systems

This chapter began with a statement that the CMHC has given much that it promised, but to relatively few. The fact that its achievements have been more qualitative than quantitative does not alter the fact that the CMHC has contributed significantly to an improved approach, within a clinical frame of reference, to the treatment of the mentally ill. In this connection, it is well to bear in mind that of the five essential services mandated by the initial CMHC legislation, four (inpatient, outpatient, partial hospitalization, and emergency) are strictly clinical; and the fifth (consultation and education to community agencies) has a strong clinical component if it is interpreted as this author believes it was intended to be. Thus it is fairer to measure the achievements of the CMHC by the criteria imposed in the initial mandate than by those superimposed by subsequent misinterpretations of parts of the mandate.

As Wachspress points out,[18] the concept in activation of the CMHC represented a tremendous advance in psychiatric care, especially as this approach was able to make treatment programs accessible locally and with reasonable immediacy. Even if the promise of full integration of fragmented services has not been entirely realized, an effective approach to improved continuity of care has at least been set in motion. The CMHC was able to identify patients with schizophrenia. Either on the basis of identification of troubled individuals by others in the community, or by the presence of unusual behavior patterns, the health care system affords another possible entry for the patient with this illness; many patients with schizophrenia and other emotional illnesses present vague medical problems at the onset. A decentralized, local, accessible medical service should be a gain rather than a loss in the recognition of serious psychiatric illness. It is important that those features of the CMHC which made treatment possible be maintained. These include easy availability and access of care (geographical decentralization and 24-hour services) and the mobilization of community resources which should continue to be possible in the emerging ambulatory care component of the health care system.

CMHCs, both urban and rural, have pioneered in their efforts to make services accessible to all consumers. In urban settings, this has been accomplished largely by the use of local neighborhood facilities—churches, public buildings, or rented storefronts. In rural areas, traveling teams have gone to local communities and made themselves available within the community itself. In both circumstances, but particularly the urban areas, the mental health neighborhood facility could easily be expanded into a primary health care facility. Space is usually available, consumers are already involved at the point of primary care delivery, and most important, potential users already are establishing a pattern of seeking service. Just as these local facilities now link with other components of the health care system (day hospitals, inpatient units), so linkage with secondary and tertiary health care facilities should be accomplished without great difficulty. A shared facility would enable the medical component to have available to it the community information of the mental health center and some of the trust that hopefully has been accorded the mental health center. The mental health center itself would be strengthened by these additional care-giving components.

Continuity of care within the mental health center must occupy a central position in the general health care delivery system. One could argue that it is more difficult to maintain continuity of care for people who are mentally ill than for those with physical illnesses. The techniques developed for providing continuity of care in the mental health field, such as home visiting when patients fail to keep appointments, are transferable to the health care system. Indeed, it is desirable if not essential that the mental health approach be built into this system. The two systems at the local delivery points are certainly more similar than different. An incorporation with general medical services is not an abrogation of responsibility of the community mental health approach, but rather a return to its original, essentially medical, mandate. Moreover, early detection of mental illness will be facilitated through the earlier detection of its manifestations as first seen by the family physician or the pediatrician.

PARAPROFESSIONAL PERSONNEL

The community mental health approach, in demanding decentralization of services, precipitated a need for developing interrelationships with locally based groups. That the employment of persons with local roots would serve this need was perceived quite early in CMHC history. In many cases, such persons had little, if any, occupational training, and were employed at nonprofessional levels, usually clerical. However, their ability to fill another need soon became apparent: the need for better understanding of the social matrix from which the CMHC's patients were emerging. Increasing numbers of indigenous persons began to be employed and trained as paraprofessional mental health workers. This movement preceded and presaged the major movement now developing in the general health care system toward paraprofessional manpower development. The implications of the movement are profound, in respect both to opening up new possibilities for communications among people of different backgrounds, and to optimum utilization of human resources. The development of paraprofessional manpower hence must be regarded as among the CMHC's unequivocal contributions to all human caretaking endeavors.

IMPLICATIONS FOR TRAINING

The CMHCs interest in the social environment of its patients, its insistence on viewing the individual as a functioning member of a family and of a larger societal group, and its emphasis on accessibility and continuity of care are all relevant to contemporary developments in medical (including psychiatric) training. Although episodic treatment still generally characterizes the health care system and its training facilities, strenuous efforts are being made to enable medical students, interns, and house officers to see patients within their social context from the onset of illness to functional restoration. Within this framework of continuous care, it is possible to help the trainee become familiar with available resources and support systems. For example, he can learn how to utilize various financing sources, graduated care facilities, professional personnel other than physicians, and paraprofessional personnel.

The CMHC thus has served to rationalize a developing approach to patient care and to present the trainee with opportunities for learning the approach. In many CMHCs, these opportunities have been used. But it may be that medical educators have not used them sufficiently—at least in part because they see the

CMHC as somewhat removed from the mainstream of medical training. Another factor is the perception of the CMHC by its users as primarily a service center whose limited funds must not be diverted to training, a problem also encountered, incidentally, by neighborhood health centers. If young professionals (and this applies to all the health-related professions as well as to medicine) are to learn the important relationship between patient and community, providers and educators must somehow convince users that all three groups will have to cooperate in developing arrangements making this possible.

Who's in Charge Here?

Other problems of the health care system are clearly not advantages. Somers,[19] in a recent article entitled, "Who's in Charge Here?—or Alice Searches for a King in Mediland," highlights the administrative confusion still existing in health care systems. This underlines the dilemma which the mental health specialist faces when he sees the inevitability of merging of the two systems: When, how, and with whom? In actuality, the community psychiatrist, accustomed as he is to seeking hidden subsystems within the community, will find the medical subsystem somewhat easier to identify than others, and will quickly come to appreciate the power sources and the conflicts. Moreover, he can look increasingly to providers of payment, be they government or nongovernment insurers or vendors, to determine who is in charge of organizing the system. This search for who is in charge is familiar to all directors of community mental health centers. We have all learned, perhaps to our personal dismay, that he who is in charge of the purse strings is, in fact, in charge. The community mental health administrator is in a uniquely favorable position to make use of his hard-won knowledge as he attempts to bring about the integration of his facilities with those of the general health system.[10] He may even be able to teach the health care administrator some lessons.

REFERENCES

1. Leopold RL: Urban problems and the community mental health center: Multiple mandates, difficult choices. Background and current status. Am Orthopsychiatry 41:144–167, 1971
2. Adelberg A, Kuhn DS: Urban problems and the community mental health center: Multiple mandates, difficult choices. Administration. Presented before the annual meeting of the American Orthopsychiatric Association, San Francisco, March 1970 (unpublished).
3. Schwartz DA: Community mental health in 1972: An assessment. In Bellak L, Bart-
en HH (eds): Progress in Community Mental Health, vol II, New York, Grune & Stratton, 1972
4. Bolman WM: The mental health consortium. In Bellak L, Barten HH (eds): Progress in Community Mental Health, vol II. New York, Grune & Stratton, 1972
5. Gardner EA, Snipe JN: Toward the coordination and integration of personal health services. Am Public Health 60:2068–2078, 1970
6. Caplan G: The theory and practice of mental health consultation. In Bellak L, Barten HH (eds): Progress in Community Mental

Health, vol II. New York, Grune & Stratton, 1972

7. Freidson E: Profession of Medicine. New York, Dodd Mead, 1971

8. Freeman HE, Levine S, Reeder LG: Handbook of Medical Sociology. Englewood Cliffs, NJ, Prentice-Hall, 1972

9. Hurst JW, Walker HK: The Problem-Oriented System. New York, Medcom,1972

10. Leopold RL, Kissick WL: A community mental health center, regional medical program, and joint planning. Amer J Psychiat 126:1718–1726, 1970

11. Boulding KE: The concept of need for health services. Milbank Mem Fund Q 44:202–225, 1966

12. Roman M, Schmais A: Consumer participation and control: A conceptual overview. In Bellak L, Barten HH (eds): Progress in Community Mental Health, vol II. New York, Grune & Stratton, 1972

13. Somers AR (ed): The Kaiser-Permanente Medical Care Program: A Symposium. New York, Commonwealth Fund, 1971

14. Redd LS, Meyers ES, Scheidmondel P L: Health Insurance and Psychiatric Care, Utilization and Cost. Washington, DC, American Psychiatric Association, 1972

15. Leopold RL: The West Philadelphia Community Mental Health Consortium in retrospect: Supraprocess and infraprocess. In Greenblatt M, Sharaf MR (eds): The Dynamics of Program Development. New York, Grune & Stratton, 1971

16. Peck HB, Roman M, Kaplan SR: Community action programs and the comprehensive mental health center. In Greenblatt M, Emery PE, Glueck BC: Poverty and Mental Health. Washington, DC, American Psychiatric Association, 1967

17. Bolman WM, Goldman W: The San Francisco Westside Community Mental Health Center, Inc.: Development of mental health consortium of private agencies. In Levenson AI, Beigel A (eds): The Community Mental Health Center: Strategies and Programs. New York, Basic Books, 1972

18. Wachspress M: Goals and functions of the community mental health center. Am J Psychiat 129:187–190, 1972

19. Somers AR: Who's in charge here?—or Alice searches for a king in mediland. N Engl J Med 287:849–855, 1972

John C. Glidewell, Ph.D.

10

A Nonmedical Model for Community Mental Health

The basic idea of this essay is that there are some powerful approaches to community mental health, approaches which could well be added to traditional clinical intervention which would go far beyond the mental health center, and which would enable the mental health center to free itself from unrealistic community expectations.

At the outset I shall make some quite general assertions, as a guide to the proposals to follow. Subsequently, I shall present concrete explanations for the reasonableness of the initial assertions.

GENERAL STATEMENT

The helping dyad has been, both traditionally and currently, an enormously effective social structure for clinical intervention, but the helping dyad also has some inherent limitations. One such limitation is found in the social conflict between real community needs for highly specialized skills and real community needs for limiting the social power generated by such skills. A second limitation lies in the fact that, although the traditional helping dyad is particularly effective in correcting failures of socialization that are low in prevalence, it is quickly overloaded by more general failures of socialization that are high in prevalence.

A possible approach to mitigating community conflict and treatment overloads lies in nonclinical community facilitation of socialization, i.e., facilitation of the accomplishment of developmental tasks. Increases in the variety of cognitive and social resources actively available in the community would facilitate both cognitive and social development. Such increases in active availability could be accomplished by inventions of new system linkages in modern communities. Inventions of effective system linkages would be most stimulated by actions of small, powerful decision-making groups involved in community governance.

Successful intervention in decision-making groups requires a public professional practice of social intervention, subject to public scrutiny. The acceptance of the duty to provide for public scrutiny and accountability entitles the professional social practitioner to the right to influence (not to determine) public policy.

Following are some explanations of some concrete empirical knowledge and some rearrangements of that knowledge into a schema for a new extraclinical, extramedical approach to the facilitation of human development.

CLINICAL INTERVENTION AND COMMUNITY RESPONSE

In all sorts of societies, primitive and complex, there has been a long-standing arrangement for dealing with the individual who behaves so badly or strangely that he is considered to be ill or possessed by evil spirits. He is temporarily relieved of his usual responsibilities and assigned to a helping dyad—a temporary relationship with a person of special status who is to help him. Many helping processes take the social form of the dyad: healing, tutoring, consulting, training, confession, and exorcising. The helper is always a person of special status due to his age, knowledge, skill, or magical power: doctor, lawyer, priest, golf pro. In some patrilineal societies, the mother's brother is assigned to help her sons when they respond to their father badly or strangely.[1]

The special resources of the helper are not readily transferable to the client. To do so takes too long, or takes special aptitude, or takes aging—a process which cannot be hurried. It is either uneconomic or impossible to train the client to help himself. Very likely the special intimate social and emotional atmosphere of the dyad is necessary for the helping process to occur. It may take two to help—or even three.[2]

Historically, in nearly all cultures, the helper has been constrained by community sanction to act in accord with the best interests of his client and to return the client to his regular duties as soon as possible. But there is a most unusual license involved. Because of the special and esoteric nature of the helper's knowledge, wisdom, or magic, it is the helper who determines what is, in fact, an action in the best interest of the client. The client is relieved not only of his duty to help himself, but also of his right to determine his own best interests. He is required to undergo pain, distress, and various indignities because the helper knows what is best for him.[3]

The belief that the helper has special skills and knows—better than the client himself—what is best for the client produces an extraordinary allocation of power to the helper. The power imbalance so created is the social force that generates the great concern of the community that the special social power of the helper be kept under community control. In almost all helping dyads there is some form of privileged communication. Although the deviant is expected to expose his personal problems (or his personal devils) to his helper, he is protected from a more general exposure. Even in the most complex of privileged societies, the professional practitioner in the helping professions is rarely observed in interaction with his client. Consequently, such dyads have little systemic linkage to the regular system. Citizens have no channel of direct influence; professional colleagues have little opportunity for direct surveillance.

Another source of community control is the time limitation—the helping dyad is a temporary relationship. The time limits are intended to preclude continued exploitation. These limits also decrease the possibility of repeating mistakes. But when mistakes are made, there is more freedom from sanction. The remarkable and often unnoticed thing is that the professional practitioner is allowed to charge the client extra fees for the practitioner's mistakes. If you've ever had prescriptions changed or x-rays retaken or surgery repeated, you may have noticed that it is the client who pays for the mistakes.

The nature of the social structure of the helping dyad produces a continuing conflict for the community. On the one hand, the community wants to have the specialized resources readily available. Indeed, the community is sometimes willing to pay quite well for them. On the other hand, the community is always uneasy about the power it grants to the helper to decide what is good for his client. The conflict produces a tension level moving in cycles from a comfortable dependency to a destructive indictment. My proposition is that, now, in this society, we are moving toward the phase of destructive indictment. Both black power groups and white power groups are attacking the professional practitioner. They are accusing him of exploitation and are denying that he acts in the best interests of his clients. They demand limitations on his power to price his services, to decide who gets them, to decide who pays for them, and to judge the effectiveness of their results.[3] As for the mental health practitioner specifically, many newly powerful groups question whether there is any need at all for mental health services. "First," they say, "give us food, clothing, and safe housing."

THE CHALLENGE OF ACCOUNTABILITY

The trend is not limited to the newly powerful militants. Much more tractable community policy makers in the Establishment are engaged in an earnest and puzzling search for some form of realistic accountability to the community by the professional practitioner. Especially in community mental health, where the practitioner intervenes not just in the life of an individual, but in all the social systems of the community, the search for a realistic accountability is frustrating.

A tradition of accountability exists, but the progressive deterioration of the linkage between the health institution and the community has made the more traditional accountability nearly obsolescent. The choice of practitioner by the client grows more limited and subject more and more to conditions of proximity, limited practice, and economic means. Even the privileged client finds that he has less information that he needs to make an intelligent choice of practitioner. If you have moved to a new city recently—and the odds are good that you have—you know how hard it is to get the information you need to choose a lawyer in the new community.

State licensing is largely controlled by the professional practitioners themselves. Licensing boards have grown more rigid, traditional, and resistant to innovation. Internal professional surveillance by professional associations seems to act as often to protect the practitioner from discredit as to protect the client from exploitation. As professional associations invest more of their resources in attempts to influence public policy, the associations are seen as acting to increase the power of the practitioner, and, therefore, they are seen as acting against the public interest.

Time limits on the relationship are not yet so outmoded. Mental hospitals especially have been vigorously involved in reducing the time the patient is in the hospital. Ironically enough, the helping relationship with the mental patient may be the one kind of relationship that the public is willing to allow to run to very long terms. Chronic problems increasingly become the problems requiring help— chronic mental illness, chronic poverty, chronic antisocial behavior, and chronic economic incompetence. As that trend continues, one may expect that the competence of the practitioner will be questioned, simply because his patients don't get better. In addition, he will be suspected of exploitation because he continues for a long period to collect his fees, whether from his patients or from a third party, while his patients continue to suffer.

As the demands for control have grown, the professional practitioners have conducted some experiments in seeking community representation in groups planning or conducting programs of professional practice. The question of who can claim to represent the community is recurrent and perplexing. There is no parliamentarian method of voting for a representative in the health institution. Even more perplexing is the question about what decisions are best based upon specialized knowledge and what decisions are best based upon a representative citizen's extraprofessional judgment about the interests of the community. This confusion regularly occurs when planning groups of practitioners and citizens ask: Who is to get the scarce services? Who is to price the services? Who is to pay for them? Who is to judge the results?

The social analyses of Loomis[4] and of Hauser[5] have made clear that as the society becomes increasingly more complex and highly specialized, accountability for the consequences of social action becomes more and more vague. Accompanying the increasing ambiguity of accountability is an increasing questioning of the goodwill of the specialist with arcane knowledge and esoteric skills, by both his clients and the community at large. As it becomes less and less possible for the client and the community to evaluate the quality of the highly specialized services received, distrust takes root and grows to cover a wider range of practitioners, from television repairmen to operators of blood banks.[6]

The discontent with and conflicts about the extraordinary social power of practitioners with esoteric skills have widely-distributed roots in the institutions of the society, but they have one root, at least, that is readily subject to change.

ILLNESS AND HUMAN DEVELOPMENT

In the course of the growth of the mental health movement, many failures to accomplish developmental tasks have been defined as illnesses. In the tenor of the times, this concept had considerable social utility. It did much to mitigate the unwise and ineffective punishment of individuals for the faults of the social systems in which they lived. It was, nevertheless, an unrealistic definition.

It was unrealistic, first, because it implied that some healing art was required for treatment, when some ingenuity in resource allocation and training methods was really more appropriate to the problem. In addition, it was unrealistic because the resources were more often devoted to changing the individual to fit social systems and less often devoted to changing the social systems to tolerate or to accommodate to individual differences. It was unrealistic in a third way also. It applied the clinical approach to phenomena of very high prevalence, even though that approach is best suited to dealing with phenomena of very low prevalence. Historical data (e.g., Duffy[7]) make it clear that the clinical approach has been immensely successful in curing many disorders—until the number of cases overloads the facilities and manpower. The clinical approach did not evolve from epidemics, nor did it evolve as a socialization device for the population.

It is enough just to point to the well-known data[8] showing how clinical facilities in mental health are now overloaded and, given current definitions of the need for treatment, are going to become more and more overloaded. Nonclinical intervention at the system level places the responsibility for facilitating the accomplishment of developmental tasks on persons and groups more competent to discharge the responsibility—the agents of socialization. Because it is a more realistic view of the problem, it makes a more realistic use of facilities and manpower. There will remain severe failures to accomplish developmental tasks due to constitutional factors or intense stress or severe deprivation—problems of low prevalence. Such problems are appropriately treated by clinical methods and can be so managed without overloading that care-offering system.

An important clarification and explication can be derived from a consideration of the available data relevant to failures to accomplish developmental tasks.

The ideas are based upon knowledge available from the research of diverse scientists who never intended that their findings be put together as a basis for preventive social intervention. I shall propose, however, that it is possible to organize these findings so as to formulate a tentative schema that will serve as a guide for an extraclinical preventive social intervention. If such intervention is carefully observed and analyzed, the tentative schema will become a guide to the creation of new and sounder knowledge as a basis for yet more effective preventive social intervention. Who could oppose such a noble purpose?

DEVELOPMENTAL TASKS

The concept of "stage" in human development has been subjected to a wide variety of tests over a long period of time by, for example, Freud,[9] Gesell,[10] Erikson,[11] and Piaget.[12] The findings show that the human organism grows through a series of stages, each having its sequential developmental tasks. The sequence of the stages is quite similar for persons living in diverse cultures. Failure to accomplish the tasks at one stage of development limits the approach to, and reduces the resources available for, accomplishing the tasks of later stages. On the other hand, mastery of the tasks at one stage of development enhances the approach to, and increases the resources available for, accomplishing the tasks of the next stages. "Development," i.e., the gain in reaching a "higher" stage, is conceived to be a gain in differentiation, integration, and complexity—all leading to an increased adaptability to changing environments. Against this background, childhood is a critical period of development, not because there is any fixation of psychosocial problems during childhood, but because during childhood there remain more subsequent stages to be influenced, positively and negatively, by the accomplishment of current development tasks.

As a corollary to these propositions, any lag in the accomplishment of developmental tasks becomes greater with age, a phenomenon of accumulated deficit. Similarly, there are some points in the process which may be critical periods, in that a given stage must be reached by the end of the period if it is to be reached at all.[13]

The concept of staging in human development is an old one, but let Piaget's work stand as an excellent example. The movement from one stage to the next is conceived to be a categorical, qualitative change in the kinds of processes included in behavior, thinking, feeling. In cognitive development, the change is located in the structure or schemata of thought processes; in social development, the change is located in the structure or schemata of the processes of support and control of individual behavior by others. Kohlberg[14] found cognitive development to be a necessary but not a sufficient condition for moral development.

Stages follow each other in an invariant sequence; cultural objects, beliefs, symbols may accelerate or retard movement from one stage to the next, but they do not change the sequence. For example, Kohlberg[15] reported identical sequences of moral development in boys in the United States, Great Britain, Taiwan, Yucatan, and Turkey. Each stage is, in addition, a necessary but not a sufficient condition for advancement to the next. Both Hunt[16,17] and Bloom[18] have shown that failure to accomplish the tasks of one stage limits the accomplishment of the tasks of the following stages.

The key concept used to explain the transition from one stage to the next is conflict—conflict between what a person expects and what a person experiences. Such conflicts motivate the person to shift his attention, to perceive aspects of the situation which he did not notice before, and to center his attention on some new dimension of a percept. From such shifting or "decentration" new processes are included in the behavior, thinking, and feeling of the person, and new schemata are generated. *Voilà!* A new stage of development has arrived.

All the foregoing lead to the critical element for social intervention. Experience is essential to development; more or richer stimulation leads to movement, a more broadly and deeply secured movement, from one stage to the next. More specifically, the wider the variety of stimuli, the greater is the facilitation of the accomplishment of developmental tasks. But variety is not enough. The variety must lead to conflict between expectation and experience and thus to decentration and accommodation. In that sense, the alternative stimuli must be nearly equivalent in the capacity to generate conflict, decentration, and accommodation.

Based upon the foregoing, if social intervention is to facilitate psychosocial development, it must extend the variety of conflict-inducing psychosocial resources acting upon a person. In addition, however, social intervention must provide mechanisms for managing the tensions accompanying the conflict induced by unexpected experiences, so that the outcome is a developmental change and not some distortion or denial of the new experience.

NICHE BREADTH AND EXPLORATORY BEHAVIOR

There is a key assumption in the proposition that environmental variety facilitates development. The assumption is that the organism will come into contact with and cope with the variety of resources made available.[19]

It is a fascinating experience to observe a child who has been introduced to a strange room containing a variety of dark doors leading to unknown new areas and a variety of lighter doors leading to partly visible new areas. Some children find a comfortable position—or as comfortable as possible—and remain there until they can return to a familiar area. Other children begin immediately, with zest and vigor, to explore the visible area, then the partly visible areas, then the invisible areas beyond the dark doors. Indeed, a few approach the dark doors first.

The variations in exploratory behavior in children can be seen to be remarkably constant from birth to adulthood, as Chess and her associates have so well demonstrated.[20] It is also true that children from unchanging environments with little variety of stimuli tend to sit; those from changing environments with great variety of stimuli tend to explore.

Smith,[21] in his review of field ecology, has shown that increases in the variety of resources (nutrients) available will induce increases in the extent of the range over which an organism will be found. There is also the parallel finding that the extent of tolerance of the individual organism for a variety of environmental stimuli is related to the extent of the range over which the organism is found. One may conclude that environmental variety will stimulate exploratory behavior until such behavior reaches the limit of tolerance of the individual organism. This limit of tolerance may be determined by the balancing foundation of nonconflicting (assimilable) experiences, a foundation of confidence upon which the novel conflicting experiences are confronted. Hunt[16] analyzed this balance as the problem of "match." Kelly[22] addressed this problem in planning his studies of population exchange and coping behavior in high school: "Work on the joint evolution of habitat selection and niche breadth, on the role of productivity of biotic environments, and on food-getting procedures, all converge in supporting the theorem that environmental uncertainty (randomness) leads to increased niche breadth.''

The social analogy to the exploration of space is the exploration of role or role-taking behavior. To take the role of the other, even in one's imagination, is an exploration. In addition, the exploration leads to conflict between expectations and experience as often as the interests of the other are perceived to be in conflict with one's own interests.

Feffer[23] has developed an integration of the constructs of Asch and Piaget which explicates social development as the process of resolution of conflicts engendered by exploratory role taking. In the simplest sense, the resolution follows the dialectic. Polarities (thesis-antithesis) of social roles are reconstructed in some broader or deeper concept (synthesis) which includes the original polarities but within a more general and more compelling complementary interdependence. For example, the powerful social agent, or father figure, is first seen as the oppressor of the needs of the actor. When, however, one can "put oneself" in the place of the powerful social agent, even in imagination, one sees that the powerful agent also must make resources available to the less powerful and he must regularly risk making mistakes which discredit the base of his power, whether expertise, social position, or control of rewards. Similarly, the less powerful actor receives valued resources in exchange for his compliance and is relieved of the risks of making mistakes. The broader concept of a complementary exchange of power for resources and risk taking is a new schema—a synthesis. The classic socialization constructs are thus seen in the theory. However explained in specific role relationships, the wider the variety of opportunity for, and the wider the variety of models available for, role taking, the greater the facilitation of the accomplishment of psychosocial developmental tasks.

The immediate objective of social intervention, then, is to induce conflict between expectation and experience. An increase in the variety of environmental stimuli—cognitive or social—can be expected to induce such conflicts up to some limit of tolerance, a limit determined by the balance of assimilation possibilities and accommodation demands.

TURNOVER AND SYSTEM LINKAGE

To imagine how to increase the variety of stimulation in an environment, one looks to ''natural'' processes which provide variety, a stimulation to explore, and a floor of assimilative constancy as a basis for foresight. Hauser has said:

Man is the only culture-building animal on the globe. He not only adapts to environment, he creates environment to which to adapt, and he is still trying to learn to live in the world that he himself has created—a world of large populations, great densities, and great population diversification subject to rapid technological and social change. It is within this perspective that we can better understand the physical problems of the United States— air and water pollution, traffic congestion, parking problems and the commuter crisis; the personal and social problems of juvenile delinquency, crime and drug addiction, the revolt of the younger generation . . .; the problems of intergroup relations climaxed by the Negro revolt; and the problems of governance on the Federal, state, and local levels.[24]

Haire's analyses[25] have shown that as social systems increase in size and density, the members have greater and more varied human resources available to them, but they have more trouble using the resources. Both Indik[26,27] and Thomas and Fink[28] have found that an increase in size and density tends to be followed by a greater centralization of social power. Slater found a faster evolution of more highly specialized roles,[29] and Asch[30] and others[31] a greater demand for conformity. Larger systems provide more opportunities to participate but stimulate less participation. Larger systems provide central roles in fewer activities and less assimilation of decisions made.[27,30–32] In larger systems there is a greater resource input but a smaller demand for resources.[33]

Complexity of social organization is a concomitant of both increased size and specialization of tasks. The advantages of both large and small size might be obtained if the larger system were organized into subsystems with active linkages. Social forces inherent in small groups provide both the demand and the opportunity for intimacy, identification, and conformity—the foundation of assimilative experiences necessary for personal security. The larger, fast-changing suprasystem provides the population exchange, the variety of resources, the unexpected experiences—the conflicts necessary for psychosocial development. The key, however, lies in the linkages among the components of the community. Communities are systems of groups which tend to hold intergroup suspicions, to reduce communication between groups, and to reduce the rate of interaction and interchange of resources between groups, as shown so clearly in the experiments of Sherif[34] and Deutsch[35] and in the interpretations of Loomis.[4]

The fact is that the variety is already present, generated by the rapid increase in size, density, mobility, and complexity. The inventions, technical and social, become encapsulated in subsystems poorly linked to, or indeed estranged from, other subsystems. As illustrated by the work of Mansfield,[36,37] introduction of innovations is relatively quick in large organizations, relatively slower in smaller ones. The diffusion of innovations, however, is relatively slow in larger organizations; relatively fast in smaller ones. It follows, then, that the stimulation of environmental variety in a society undergoing rapid increases in size, density, mobility, and complexity, is powerfully mediated by linkages among the subsystems in the society and the interchange of resources channeled through such linkages.

Traditionally, system linkages take a variety of forms.[38] The most obvious and extensive form is mass communication.[39] As the impact of mass communication is felt more clearly, a greater variety of resources will become available to, and *have an impact upon*, the conflicts between expectation and experience, by modifying expectations while experiences remain constant. Mass communication has enormous scope; it has limited intensity.

The most intense of linking devices is the traditional arrangement of overlapping roles, and the traditional context for the linkage was the neighborhood. In the older, traditional neighborhood the health agent served on the school board, teachers served in churches, clergymen were on village councils, businessmen raised funds for welfare agencies. All of them met in grocery stores, drug stores, and street celebrations. The device of overlapping roles has limited scope, but it has great intensity. Traditional neighborhoods, however, have become diluted in solidarity, diffuse in norms, and sporadic in interaction; they no longer provide a context for linkage. As well developed by students of community power structure, the overlapping role is, however, still a powerful linkage device at the broader community level.

Related to the device of overlapping role is the role of the opinion leader. E. M. Rogers[40] has shown how opinion leaders are key influences on the diffusion of innovations. Katz and Lazarsfeld[41] found them to be critical in the modification of political behavior. Opinion leaders evolve more or less spontaneously, have high intensity, and often have considerable scope of activity. They represent an especially potent device for facilitation of development.

Detached workers and satellite groups, detached from one subsystem and assigned to another, are particularly useful where expertise as well as intensity are required. The scope is limited. Maintenance crews, detached from an equipment supplier to a large customer, have worked well in industry. Detached units are most powerful when representing a large group of consumers to the purveyors of some community service. The current attraction to the use of indigenous workers in health agencies is a well-known example of workers or satellite groups detached from the larger community to represent it in a service-providing subsystem.[42] In the opposite direction, the detachment of the group worker to cope with juvenile gangs is a familiar example of a linking device requiring expertise, intensity, but limited scope. The limitation of scope has been the major objection to the detached worker in large urban slums. In addition, the risk of a shift of loyalty (of "going native") has always accompanied detached units and workers.

What is required, then, is further social invention of linking mechanisms. The linkages will provide the channels of interchange for the already existing variety of cognitive and social stimuli abroad in a land of rapidly increasing size, mobility, density, and complexity.

The individual is especially influenced by the nature of the social systems in which he finds himself—family, peer group, neighborhood, school, church, work place. The family has been the traditional point of entry, but the evidence is clear that the family is markedly limited by the larger systems in which the members live. Miller and Riessman[43] have demonstrated those influences in the working classes. Pettigrew[44] has made clear the community limitations on black families. The same social forces, if not the same deprivations, limit the actions in middle-class families.

As points of entry for the invention of system linkages, larger community systems are more promising. Especially important are those small groups of powerful adults whose decisions so greatly influence the allocation of resources to community institutions. Changes in the decision-making processes in such groups have potentially broad consequences on the human development of many people.

Generally, it has been demonstrated that the decision-making processes of small groups can be modified. Merton[45] has shown how small decision-making groups are norm-setting and norm-enforcing reference groups. On the other hand, a remarkable series of experiments by Lewin and his students[46,47] has shown that small groups are also instruments for social change.[48,49] The outcome of the experiments can be summarized as follows: (1) group discussion of controversial proposals usually makes explicit some latent conflicts between cultural values and social norms;[39,41] (2) group support of valued innovation is increased by the explicit *individual* decision (public or private) to adopt the innovation;[50,51] (3) social inventions are supported by the perception that a large number of other group members are committed to experiment with the social invention;[50] and (4) any behavior change is best supported by a group leadership which exercises only reward power (as opposed to coercive power).[49,52]

As yet, nobody has consciously tried the method, but it seems altogether reasonable that small groups of powerful persons in community institutions—political, economic, health, judicial, religious, educational, industrial—are potent sources of social inventions of systems linkages in modern urban communities. Indeed, the guide for the intervention has been set out by Lewin's students: Present the decision makers with some problem involving conflicts between values and norms concerning system linkages or lack of them. Collaborate in generating a wide variety of ideas about the costs and rewards of experimenting with novel linkages. Seek individual and group commitment to implement inventive, experimental social linkages.

While Lewin and his students demonstrated that social intervention can have consequences, they also demonstrated that it is rife with unexpected consequences. If the professional practitioner is to accept the obligation for accountability, his social interventions must be kept under careful surveillance. The unexpected consequences must be quickly known and modifications in approaches quickly made—often capitalizing on unexpected consequences as variety-inducing events. The real lesson of Lewin's use of action research is that experimental social intervention can, by the development of active feedback loops, become a self-developing process. Not only is the variety of stimuli increased in the interest of individual development, the variety of social structures is increased for community development.

Indeed, the development of active new feedback loops is as sharp a challenge for social invention as is the development of new system linkages. Methods for collecting reliable and valid data are becoming more readily available and unobtrusive. The development of composite indexes of success in accomplishing developmental tasks in whole populations is well under way. Something like a psychosocial "cost-of-living index" is probably feasible. Sheldon and Moore[53] have collected highly sophisticated evaluations of social indicators in almost every community institution and point out the possible forms of new indicators. Bellak[54] has made some provocative suggestions for a new index of adaptation in a community.

Research designs to provide rigorous inferences from social intervention data are already available, even if seldom employed. Campbell,[55] especially, has designed time series studies that, even post hoc, provide rigor and precision in judging the impact of social interventions. Media for direct, two-way communication between the public and the practitioner are available here and now.

Under these conditions, practitioners involved in community affairs ought firmly to accept an old obligation. Whether guided by such an amalgam as is proposed here or by some other construct about the promise of social intervention, a professional practitioner in community affairs should be guided by some concept of what he is doing. He should also be committed to close public scrutiny of what he is doing. The privacy of private practice is unassailable; the openness of public practice is just evolving. I am proposing a limited ethic: (1) the social practitioner should have a clear idea about what he is doing and should be willing and able to articulate it clearly on demand; (2) the social practitioner should submit his work to close public scrutiny. The two obligations imply that a practitioner should be always ready to join in any collaborative attempt to compare what he is observed to do with what he intended to do. In the interests of science, one can expect that the store of knowledge about the nature of social systems will be significantly increased by carefully observed attempts to intervene in them. In the interests of a realistic and just society, one can expect that clearly evaluated experiences will provide a firmer base for both a reasoned stability and a realistic social change.[56]

Given the assumption of an obligation for accountability, the social practitioner may find it appropriate to begin to exercise a new right—the right to try to influence public policy. The social practitioner ought to use the body of empirical knowledge available to him to make rational extrapolations from that knowledge and his experiences. Based on such extrapolations, he ought to articulate clearly his views of the psychosocial implications of any existing or proposed public policy.

In the performance of the duty to provide accountability and in the exercise of the right to influence public policy, the practitioner will find himself in direct confrontation with agents of community institutions. Most such agents will distrust the practitioner's goodwill, perceive a conflict of interests with the practitioner, and seek relief through some form of political power. The resolution of such social conflicts can lead to broader and deeper conceptions of the great variety of resources being exchanged and modified in the relationship. Resolution can lead to a discovery of deeply invested complementary resources in each of the roles—practitioner and citizen—and a reciprocity of interchange which is at least temporarily just and equitable.

REFERENCES

1. Freilich M: The natural triad in kinship and complex systems. Am Sociol Rev 29:529–540, 1964
2. Glidewell JC: A social psychology of men-
tal health. In Golann S, Eisdorfer C (eds). Handbook of Community Mental Health. New York, Appleton, 1972
3. Glidewell JC: The professional practitioner

and his community. Chairman's address delivered at the annual meeting of the Mental Health Section, American Public Health Association, Detroit, Nov 12, 1968

4. Loomis CP: In praise of conflict and its resolution. Am Sociol Rev 32:875–890, 1967

5. Hauser PM: The chaotic society. Am Sociol Rev 34:1–19, 1969

6. Glidewell JC: Priorities for psychologists in community mental health. In Rosenblum G (ed): Issues in Community Psychology and Preventive Mental Health. Report of the Task Force on Community Mental Health, Division 27, American Psychological Association. New York, Behavioral Publications, 1971

7. Duffy J: A History of Public Health in New York City, 1625–1866. New York, Russell Sage, 1968

8. Arnhoff FN, Rubinstein EA, Speisman JC (eds): Manpower for Mental Health. Chicago, Aldine, 1969

9. Freud S: A General Introduction to Psychoanalysis. New York, Liveright, 1935

10. Gesell A: Infancy and Human Growth. New York, Macmillan, 1928

11. Erikson EH: Childhood and Society. New York, Norton, 1950

12. Piaget J: The Origins of Intelligence in Children. New York, Norton, 1952

13. Langer J, Kuhn D: Relations between logical and moral development. In Kohlberg L, Turiel E (eds): Recent Research in Moral Development. New York, Holt, 1971

14. Kohlberg L: The development of modes of moral thinking and choice in the years ten to sixteen. Unpublished PhD dissertation, University of Chicago, 1958

15. Kohlberg L: The concepts of developmental psychology as the central guide to education: Examples from cognitive, moral, and psychological education. In Reynolds MC (ed): Proceedings of the Conference on Psychology and the Process of Schooling in the Next Decade: Alternative Conceptions. Washington DC, Bureau for Educational Personnel Development, US Office of Education, 1972

16. Hunt JMcV: Intelligence and Experience. New York, Ronald Press, 1961

17. Hunt JMcV: Toward the prevention of incompetence. In Carter J W (ed): Research Contributions from Psychology to Community Mental Health. New York, Behavi-

oral Publications, 1968

18. Bloom BS: Stability and Change in Human Characteristics. New York, Wiley, 1964

19. Barker RG: Ecological Psychology. Stanford, Stanford University Press, 1968

20. Chess S, Thomas A, Birch HG: Your Child Is a Person. New York, Viking, 1965

21. Smith RL: Ecology and Field Biology. New York, Harper & Row, 1966

22. Kelly JG: Toward an ecological conception of preventive intervention. In Carter JW (ed): Research Contributions from Psychology to Community Mental Health. New York, Behavioral Publications, 1968

23. Feffer M: Developmental analysis of interpersonal behavior. Psychol Rev 77:197–214, 1970

24. Hauser PM: After the riots, what? Univ Chicago Mag 60:4–10, 1968

25. Haire M: Biological models and empirical histories of the growth of organizations. In Haire M (ed): Modern Organizational Theory. New York, Wiley, 1959

26. Indik BP: The relationship between organization size and supervision ratio. Admin Sci Q 9:301–312, 1964

27. Indik BP: Organization size and member participation: Some empirical tests of alternative explanations. Hum Rel 18:339–350, 1965

28. Thomas EJ, Fink CF: Effects of group size. Psychol Bull 60:371–384, 1963

29. Slater PE: Role differentiation in small groups. In Hare AP, Borgatta EF, Bales RF (eds): Small Groups: Studies in Social Interaction. New York, Knopf, 1965

30. Asch SE: Studies of independence and conformity: A minority of one against a unanimous majority. Psychol Monog 70, 1956

31. Barker RG, Gump PV: Big School, Small School. Stanford, Stanford University Press, 1964

32. Hare AP: A study of interaction and consensus in different sized groups. Am Sociol Rev 17:261–267, 1952

33. Bales RF, Borgatta EF: Size of group as a factor in the interaction profile. In Hare AP, Borgatta EF, Bales RF (eds): Family, Socialization, and Interaction Process. Glencoe, Ill, Free Press, 1955

34. Sherif M, Harvey OJ, White BJ, Hood WR, Sherif CW: Intergroup Conflict and Cooperation. Norman, Okla, Institute of

Group Relations, University of Oklahoma, 1961

35. Deutsch M: Conflicts: Productive and destructive. J Soc Issues 25:7–41, 1969

36. Mansfield E: Entry, Gibrat's law, innovation, and the growth of firms. Am Econ Rev 52:1023–1051, 1962

37. Mansfield E: Intrafirm rates of diffusion of an innovation. Rev Econ Statist 45:348–359, 1963

38. Litwak E, Meyer HJ: The school and the family: Linking organizations and external primary groups. In Lazarsfeld PF, Sewell WH, Wilensky HL: The Uses of Sociology. New York, Basic Books, 1967

39. Klapper JT: The Effects of Mass Media. Glencoe, Ill, Free Press, 1961

40. Rogers EM: Diffusion of Innovations. New York, Free Press, 1962

41. Katz E, Lazarsfeld P: Personal Influence. Glencoe, Ill, Free Press, 1955

42. Reiff R, Riessman F: The indigenous nonprofessional: A strategy of change in community action and community mental health programs. Comm Mental Health J Monogr no. 1, 1965

43. Miller SM, Riessman F: The working class subculture: A new view. Soc Problems 9:86–97, 1961

44. Pettigrew TE: A Profile of the Negro American. Princeton, NJ, Van Nostrand, 1964

45. Merton RK: Social Theory and Social Structure. Glencoe, Ill, Free Press, 1957

46. Lewin K: Group decision and social change. In Swanson GE, Newcomb TM,

Hartley EL (eds): Readings in Social Psychology. New York, Holt, 1952

47. Lippitt R, Watson J, Westley B: The Dynamics of Planned Change. New York, Harcourt, 1958

48. Cartwright D: Achieving change in people: Some applications of group dynamics theory. Hum Rel 4:381–392, 1951

49. Coch L, French JRP: Overcoming resistance to change. Hum Rel 1:512–532, 1948

50. Bennett LB: Discussion, decision, commitment, and consensus in "group decision." Hum Rel 8:251–274, 1955

51. Schachter S, Hall R: Group derived restraints and audience persuasion. Hum Rel 5:397–406, 1952

52. Kipnis D: The effects of leadership style and leadership power upon the inducement of an attitude change. J Abnorm Soc Psychol 57:173–180, 1958

53. Sheldon EB, Moore WE: Indicators of Social Change. New York, Russell Sage, 1968

54. Bellak L: Community mental health and the state of the nation. In Barten HH, Bellak L (eds): Progress in Community Mental Health. New York, Grune & Stratton, 1972

55. Campbell DT: Reforms as experiments. Am Psychol 24:409–429, 1969

56. Glidewell JC: New psychosocial competence, social change, and tension management. In Carter JW (ed): Research Contributions from Psychology to Community Mental Health. New York, Behavioral Publications, 1968

William M. Bolman, M.D.

11
Policy Aspects of Citizen Participation

Consumers and the representatives of the consumers being served must both share in the decision-making processes governing the development of new organizations for the delivery of health care and in determining the priorities to be assigned to the services offered. . . . The principle of such participation marks a drastic departure from tradition and poses a host of new challenges to leaders. Nevertheless, if it is not accepted, the organization cannot succeed for lack of local confidence and support; this is particularly true of community mental health centers in inner city areas.[1]

The reader who has reached this part of the book has likely marveled over the range of structures, programs, and special needs that has been presented. A logical question should be: Who decides what happens, given this complex mix? There has been surprisingly little discussion of this issue in the psychiatric literature. The major reason is probably because it was never perceived as a problem! As long as a psychiatrist was in the picture, it was assumed that he was the one who either made the decisions or took the leadership in making them. This was certainly the case prior to the emergence of the community mental health center. The major settings in which psychiatric services were then delivered were the psychiatrist's office or a mental hospital. In either case they were mostly psychiatrist-controlled. This is reasonable since most of the decisions that had to be made were treatment decisions. Other types of decisions, such as who should be treated or who pays for treatment, were mostly made before the patient appeared at the delivery site. Thus, neither psychiatrists nor their patients paid much attention to the area, and mental health policy mostly involved the American Psychiatric Association and the National Association for Mental Health up to the late 1940s. However, the growing number of patients in mental hospitals ("one out of every two beds") and the shocking conditions of most of the hospitals led to increasing public awareness and concern. This concern inevitably resulted in more people becoming involved in mental health decisions, with a corresponding increase in the importance of mental health policy. Unfortunately, this importance has still not been reflected in the psychiatric literature, and the best discussion of mental health policy is by a sociologist, David Mechanic.[2]

Reflecting the growing importance of who makes mental health decisions was the Joint Commission on Mental Illness and Health and the recommendations assembled in its report, *Action for Mental Health*.[3] Those who were involved will recall the intense competition and political infighting that developed among different professions due to different beliefs about the nature of the problem and what should be done about it. This became especially intense as the report of the joint commission was not regarded with favor by the executive branch, for both fiscal and philosophical reasons. Thus it is hardly a secret that the resulting legislation, the Community Mental Health Centers and Mental Retardation Acts of 1963 and 1964, was bitterly opposed by many psychiatrists who felt that efforts should be concentrated in the mental hospitals and under the control of psychiatrists. Instead, what emerged was a public health psychiatric bill creating a network of mental health centers responsible to geographically defined communities. The aim of these centers was to provide a wide range of ambulatory services directed toward reducing the role of the mental hospital. The implications for the mental health professions, especially psychiatry, have been radical. Not only have psychiatrists had to share in the decision-making process, but in many instances their voice was not the dominant one. This is not really all that surprising. What had happened was that the scope of decision making had become greatly increased. The decisions that had to be made were no longer just treatment decisions, but included issues such as financing and the allocation of scarce and expensive professional resources. In fact, one can make a good case that to avoid conflict of interest psychiatrists should not have the primary say in such decisions.

In any event, passage of the Community Mental Health Centers Act of 1963 (Public Law 88-164) created a new type of mental health care delivery structure with a new set of goals, charged with a much greater scope of activity, and responsible to a geographically defined community. However, the language of the act and its application left most of the decisional authority in the hands of psychiatrists. Therefore it has taken some years of experience and conflict for the policy implications for psychiatry in community mental health centers to be felt, as witness the opening quotation from an American Psychiatric Association task force.

The result of having a psychiatrist as director and leader in the newly formed centers was as follows: In a few instances it led to the creation of innovative community programs oriented toward prevention and community involvement. In a few others it led to flagrant abuse by private practice entrepreneurs. Between these extremes, it seemed clear that the average psychiatrist's view of community mental health mostly stressed the application of individual psychotherapy to well-motivated poor people under proper psychiatric supervision. No one doubted this was good, but many questioned whether it was good enough. Psychiatrists were

simply not trained in making the complex public health and administrative decisions with which they were confronted. Further, the concepts of "community"
were not well understood by a mobile group whose affiliations tended to be
profession-based rather than neighborhood-based. And finally, psychiatric treatment
for people who were black (or other minority), poor, unmotivated, or otherwise
different was poorly understood.

The inevitable result of this series of poor fits between what was needed and
what was available has been a constant conflict over who calls the shots. This was
recognized by Howe, who documented beautifully how psychiatrists were "unfit
by virtue of being fit with an unfit fitness."[4] The degree of unfitness is most
marked between the average well-educated, affluent, white psychiatrist and people
in our central cities. Here one could define a pscyhiatrist as "a suburban carpet-
bagger who makes a living off the sufferings of the poor."

Whether or not this is a fair description of the view of psychiatry in the ghetto, it is in the central city that the struggle over who makes decisions is the most
intense and the issues presented in the clearest relief. Policy, politics, and police
have similar origins. Who makes decisions, how they are made, and how they are
enforced have always been critical societal functions. This is equally true in the
mental health center. Given the extent of central-city problems, the scarcity of
helping resources, and the disagreements over possible solutions, the central-city
community mental health center may be looked at as the most interesting and important psychiatric delivery system presently in existence. Similarly, who makes
decisions in such centers is a fascinating and instructive issue for community mental health. Therefore, this chapter focuses especially on policy making in the urban
(ghetto, central-city) community mental health center.

To begin, here are three quotations from experienced community mental
health practitioners accenting different facets of the problem:

> Wherever its location, any center will find its resources inadequate to meet directly all
> the mental health needs of its community. A center that attempts to provide every kind of
> service to every person faces the certainty of failure; a center that attempts to provide token
> service to every person risks dissipating its resources; a center that attempts to channel its
> resources to only a few, faces the dilemma of choice. Priorities will in any event be set
> for a center. The only open question is whether or not they will be *implicit* and determined
> by the capricious forces of day-to-day pressures for service or *explicit* and determined by
> a rational assessment of needs and resources with appropriate weight given to the interests
> of various groups with a stake in the matter.[5]

> Although our group initially programmed for general psychiatric disorders, we felt the
> pull towards the high visibility problems of juvenile crime, unemployment, alcoholism and
> addiction, geriatrics, and mental retardation. It led some to wish we had planned originally
> for these high visibility problems and it led others to frustration since few of these visibility
> problems are "attractive" or "responsive" to the psychiatric and parapsychiatric profes-
> sions.[6]

> In ghetto communities and economically marginal areas they [hospitals, etc.] have
> been massively insensitive to the cares of the population they were ostensibly designed to

serve, and in general, they have been maintained as fiefdoms ruled by professional, political and economic elites.[7]

In addition to these pointed comments regarding the importance of who decides mental health center policy, recent experience tells us that matters have been partly taken out of our hands. Hospitals, clinics, and mental health centers in the ghetto have found themselves invaded, picketed, or otherwise confronted by articulate and militant citizen's groups demanding a say about programs that are supposed to help them but that are designed by other people who don't live in the ghetto. This is what is meant by citizen participation and in particular, community control—better control of one's destiny. In two recent introductory articles on community control of the community mental health center, I discussed the rationale and background of the broad social movement of citizen participation that emerged between the 1950s and the present. I argued that community control was an inevitable development for many centers, and that although this shift in decisional power posed a number of problems for professionals, it was inevitable, necessary, and generally beneficial. The reasons were three: (1) to improve the effectiveness of services, (2) to correct the institutionalized racism in American psychiatry, and (3) to ensure the physical survival of ghetto hospitals, clinics, and their personnel. Those wtih further interest in the background, rationale, and an introductory bibliography of community control may wish to review these papers.[8,9] Since the present volume is oriented toward a wider audience, the remainder of this chapter discusses other aspects of citizen participation: Who are the participants? What are the issues? What types of involvement? What are the problems? What are possible solutions?

WHO ARE THE PARTICIPANTS?

The intense and dramatic manner in which citizen participation burst upon urban health and mental health care in the 1960s caused many to lose their historical perspective about this aspect of the health care delivery pattern. Citizen involvement in health matters has been a traditional part of the American pattern from the earliest days to the present via voluntary health associations, fund-raising activities, hospital board membership, and so forth. This type of voluntary activity was so normal and valuable that no one thought much about it, and physicians saw no threat to their professional prerogatives. With the advantage of hindsight, however, we can see other reasons why this was so. Hospital board members are generally successful and wealthy community members with whom physicians were pleased to associate. Similarly, voluntary health agencies tended to attract middle-class people, mostly women, who admired and cooperated with physicians in an ancillary and self-effacing role. Neither of these characterized the new citizens who wanted to participate. Instead, these new groups were usually poor, often black, and largely not college-educated. Their manner tended to be demanding, and not noticeably self-effacing, respectful, or interested in ancillary roles. Thus it was easy for physicians and other professionals to overlook the positive assets many of

Table 11-1

A Typology of People with an Interest in Community Mental Health Programs

Person	Interests
The mental health professional	A wide variety of interests and motives ranging from self-interest to technical and humanistic concerns, variously dedicated to earning a living, being helpful, treating patients, consulting, preventive efforts, etc.
Other professionals and community care givers who encounter mental health problems in their work	Assistance in making their own work easier, whether by gaining more competence (as via consultation) or by referral for treatment of needy clients
Citizens with a sense of civic obligation and a general interest in mental health	Generalized interest in being helpful, tending to be deferential to mental health professionals, especially physicians
Citizens who have encountered mental health problems, e.g., with friends, relatives, children or selves	Specialized interest, often critical, in some aspect of mental health system
Citizens who mistrust the goals or activities of mental health, generally of an ultraconservative orientation	Mostly concerned with obstructing, criticizing, and exposing so as to block mental health programs
Members of minority groups concerned with powerlessness, inequality, and unresponsive social institutions	Initially concerned with acquiring control and self-determination, then concerned with changing programs to meet minority needs

these new participants had. For example, some had acquired considerable expertise in working in community organizations and knew a great deal about the informal community structure. Others had become expert in the incredibly complex labyrinths of many public metropolitan departments involved in human services. Experience in antipoverty, civil rights, and other activities had taught ways in which one *could* fight city hall. Still others had overcome major personal obstacles (drug addiction, alcoholism, dependency, delinquency) which left them with exceptional knowledge for helping outsiders to develop treatment programs. Unfortunately, the reluctance, inexperience, and naiveté of professional groups combined with the suspicion, resentment, and newly found independence of community groups tended to create a largely adversary type of relationship. Some ways to remedy these problems are discussed in a subsequent section. By way of summary, Table 11-1 attempts to outline the major types of people who want a say in deciding how a community mental health center uses its resources. As the foregoing discussion has indicated, the only really new group is the last one. However, its influence has been enormous.

WHAT ARE THE ISSUES?

Although this is probably not a complete list, five issues stand out in making who controls a community mental health center's programs a hotly contested matter. These are ideology, conflict of priorities, money, jobs, and racism.

Ideology

This refers to basic beliefs and values about the nature of mental health and mental illness which determine what type of response, if any, is indicated.

The *conservative-liberal-radical continuum* is one dimension that every community mental health center director is familiar with. A commonly encountered conservative view is that mental disorder is basically a moral defect caused by factors such as improper self-control. It is best handled by denial, since coddling as in psychotherapy only exaggerates the lack of control. In some very conservative sectors it is noted that many psychiatrists are Jewish and have European or even Russian names, with undertones of occult Semitic and Communist conspiracies. Liberals, in contrast, believe that mental problems are like physical problems and hence should be socially recognized and accepted and treatment be made widely available. Liberals differ along the health-illness continuum, to be discussed next, but in general psychiatrists are regarded as socially valuable and respected professionals. Radicals have yet another perspective. Many believe that mental suffering is largely the result of social oppression and caused by poverty, racism, police brutality, callous welfare workers, and related forces. In this view, a psychiatrist who accepts the status quo is part of the problem, a tool of society who labels rebels as "sick" instead of combatting oppression and injustice. Since most urban communities have sizable numbers of all three types, plus mixed groups, it can readily be understood that there will be conflict over a mental health center's policies. Conservatives are encountered mostly at public gatherings, as when public funding is being sought. The well-prepared center director will treat these encounters in an equable and nondefensive way, presenting thoroughly documented statistics and cost-benefit estimates. Radicals tend to be highly visible and articulate individuals, and my experience has been that their social consciousness is much more of a help than a hindrance in community mental health work. Liberals are not always helpful, especially if they have unrecognized status and racial prejudices.

The *illness-health continuum* appears to be inevitable result of the ambiguous, multilevel, biopsychosocial nature of psychiatry/mental health. Since this ideological aspect has so many ramifications for policymaking, I have attempted to illustrate these in Table 11-2.

Experience with community mental health workers suggests that there are no clear professional divisions. Although psychiatrists tend more to be disease-oriented, and new careerists and community workers tend to be health-oriented, with social workers and psychologists variously in between, there are many divisions depending on when and where professional training occurred. One of the im-

Table 11-2

Health-Illness Ideologies in the Mental Health Field

Disease-Oriented	*Health-Oriented*
From a practical standpoint, health is best defined as the absence of disease.	Health is a positive state of well-being which includes biological, psychological, and social components.
Satisfactory measures for defining goals are vital statistics, morbidity and mortality data, disease rates, etc.	Measures for defining goals must be very broad and include data regarding malnutrition, crowding, social disorganization, distribution of diseases by geographical and ethnic factors, absence of health insurance, accessibility of health services, presence of environmental problems such as rats, lead poisoning, housing-code violations, uncollected trash.
Necessary expertise is predominantly biomedical and highly technical.	Biomedical expertise is necessary but not sufficient. Rather, knowledge of human problems and people is more important, and skills in communication and empathy are essential.
Treatment or relief of sick people is the most important activity.	Preventive programs and health monitoring with consumer involvement are of equal or more importance than treatment.
Physicians and other well-trained specialists are the key personnel; hospitals, clinics, and doctors' offices the main delivery sites.	Community organizers, mental health educators, and a wide variety of other personnel are neccessary; delivery sites must include storefront clinics and a range of community locations.
Program planning and direction are vertical with physicians and other professionals at the top of the hierarchy. Political interference is undesirable.	Planning and direction must be much more broadly based and involve horizontal policy structures. Political competition is inevitable and healthy.

plications for policymaking is that one normally finds equally good professionals with totally different ideas about how the game should be played.

Conflict of Priorities

This is listed separately because it operates whether one is illness- or health-oriented, so wide is the scope relative to resources. An example is the treatment of "illness." Policymakers in a community mental health center have to struggle with the following, among others:

1. How many beds for inpatient services? Inpatient services require the most,
    and the most expensive, personnel, thus creating the greatest demand on
    professional resources. They have no effect on the development of new cases
    of mental illness and little effect on the rehabilitative success of inpatient
    care. There is evidence that they are potentially replaceable by mobile crisis-
    intervention services. However all third-party payers continue to be hospital-
    oriented and reward inpatient care, and many patients, families, and doctors
    prefer the hospital as an organizational support for decompensated behavior.
2. Shall there be a limit on outpatient visits? Long-term crisis therapy? The Par-
    kinson effect is powerful and underestimated, especially in outpatient services.
    The incidence of such a well-defined condition as acute appendicitis has been
    shown to vary widely according to the availability of surgical treatment re-
    sources.[10] Consider how much greater must the Parkinson effect be in such
    poorly defined conditions as most mental disorders are! And as if this isn't
    bad enough, those attempting simply to make illness decisions must also deal
    with questions like: What about people who are ill but don't seek help? What
    kinds and how much outreach? What should be the policies regarding involun-
    tary hospitalization? What services should there be for children, the aged, al-
    coholics, addicts, delinquents, criminals?

In the case of the health, systems, or ecologic orientations, the clash of priorities is even greater. In my experience it is impossible to set consistent priorities
in either case. The constant shifts in funding, personnel, and community forces require the center to pursue multiple goals simultaneously. Robert Leopold captured
the essence well in his title, ''Urban Problems and the Community Mental Health
Center: Multiple Mandates, Difficult Choices.''[11] This poses a great problem
for every community mental health center. The scope, multiple activities, limited
resources, and overall complexity require the center to pay a great deal of time
to process or system functions, especially to communication, maintenance, and survival activities. Unfortunately the priorities for these administrative or managerial
needs are usually underappreciated and understaffed. Thus policymaking in most
centers is impaired by administrative inadequacies.

Finally, a brief comment should be added about the problem of where to draw
the line between community mental health and the rest of life's problems. Especially in ghetto mental health centers, the sources of problems are so many and
involve virtually all social institutions that many staff find themselves overwhelmed, depressed, radicalized. This then leads to ineffective use of one's own
energies, creating, as it were, an intrapsychic policy crisis!

Money

With the passage of community mental health center legislation, some
$50–$100 million a year were provided for these new programs. Especially in the
ghetto, this is an unbelievable amount of legitimate money, and the struggle over
who controls it is understandably intense. The issue is additionally heated by the

fact that the money doesn't really go very far. If one hires degree professionals to staff programs, $100,000 buys merely three to eight people, depending on the type of degree. If on the other hand one hires paraprofessionals or nonprofessionals, this much money will hire as many as 15 people. Added to this, the issue of control over money is superheated because sound *fiscal* behavior results in unsound *community* behavior. A community mental health veteran has said: "A center director who sees indigent patients is not behaving logically. . . . Economic incentives to see them are simply not there."[12]

Jobs

In my earlier paper on community control it was noted "the absence of jobs in the ghetto, particularly jobs that are meaningful, interesting or pay a living wage is virtually unimaginable to the average professional."[8] The poorly defined nature of community mental health, and its attractive goals which include "prevention" and "outreach" activities require hiring indigenous community workers. This means there will be a strong push to hire nonprofessionals and to develop nonhospital, nonmedical programs. This logical enough development obviously clashes with many of the beliefs of the existing mental health Establishment and further exacerbates the policy problems.

Racism

The power and pervasive nature of the racial issue is well appreciated by professionals who have worked in the ghetto, but the naiveté or unawareness of others is colossal and astounding. Hopefully the situation is changing, as reflected in a recently published bibliography on racism in mental health[13] and in Thomas and Sillen's book *Racism and Psychiatry.*[14] In any event, in many centers the issue of skin color is omnipresent in policy considerations. Sometimes it is largely beneficial and leads to corrective measures, as in drawing attention to the largely white clientele of centers. Also it has made black professionals so important and sought after that status relationships have been much more equalized. In other cases the racism issue is uncomfortable, especially for whites, as many have had little experience as the recipients of prejudice and discrimination. Above all, racism has so much reality and has so many unconscious manifestations (unconscious to whites, that is) that it is ever-present as an explanation for anything that goes wrong, and is thus deeply embedded in the whole range of policy issues and problems of the mental health center.

WHAT TYPES OF INVOLVEMENT?

What's in a word? "Involvement" or "participation" is undoubtedly in as an idea, but reality lies elsewhere. Three variables determine the type of involvement. Lay people (citizens, consumers, etc.), for a variety of reasons (both helpful

Table 11-3
Types of Involvement

Level	Type	Meaning
1	Manipulation	Professionals consult with citizens to gain political support and allies. No other changes are intended.
2	Therapy	Professionals, usually via someone delegated for the job, consult with client-citizens to help them become "less alienated."
3	Informing	Professionals meet with cooperative citizen representatives to inform them of plans, problems, and needs in order to maintain support.
4	Consultation	Professionals meet with a variety of citizen representatives to ask their advice about plans, problems, and needs.
5	Placation	Professionals meet with militant citizen representatives to prevent them from obstructing plans.
6	Partnership	Professionals and all kinds of citizens participate equally in making plans, solving problems, and meeting needs.
7	Delegated power	Professionals relinquish control of one or more specific programs to a community group.
8	Citizen control	Professionals work as employees under the direction of a citizen board.

and otherwise), want a share in making decisions about how the mental health cetner deploys its staff. Professionals variously support, question, or oppose such involvement. Organizational structures and legislative sanction vary greatly in their permissiveness for such input.

To give an overview of the varieties of outcome that may occur from this mix, Table 11-3 presents a hierarchy of citizen participation in making policy that agrees with my experience. This hierarchy is adapted from Arnstein,[15] who characterizes levels 8 to 6 as involving genuine citizen power, levels 5 to 3 as involving degrees of tokenism, and levels 2 and 1 as nonparticipation. It will be noted immediately that the observable types of public professional-community interaction are heavily weighted toward nonpartication and token relationships. Indeed, it is embarrassing and/or exasperating to observe the degree of both conscious and unconscious condescension exhibited by well-meaning professionals in trying to deal with the new citizen groups. If one recalls the ethnic and class differences of the participants again, the reason for the exclusion from sharing in power and policymaking becomes evident. For example, the majority of private hospitals and health agencies throughout the country operate as nonprofit corporations, frequently sectarian in origin, in which the organization is run by those who use it, that is at level 7 or 8. On the other hand, control of health services in the cities is far removed from those who use them. This type of policy structure is in effect an oligarchy or aristocracy, characterized by professional dominance. Indeed the struggle between this and a more democratic policy structure has been characteristic of United States history from its beginnings to the present. Alinsky, in an extremely perceptive discussion of this topic observed: "Basically our problem is still the central issue of the debate in the Federalist Papers as to whether or not the people can be trusted."[16]

Fortunately, there have been a number of developments that suggest that consumers and citizens are at least as helpful and responsible in weighing policy alternatives as professionals and other providers. In my own experience, the reason for this appears to be that the citizen/consumer has fewer vested interests and less to lose, hence can look at alternative programs with greater objectivity. Similarly, an American Medical Association Committee on Health Care of the Poor reports: "In no project were consumers telling providers how to deliver the technical aspects of medical care."[17]

Despite these indications that community/citizen/consumer control is no threat in private hospitals and suburban sites and appears to be nonthreatening in technical aspects of health care delivery, the nontechnical aspects (power, status, race) are such strong determinants of human behavior that the struggle over who controls public sector and ghetto programs will almost certainly be a major community mental health issue in the present decade. Therefore, it is important to look at the problems.

WHAT ARE THE PROBLEMS?

The discussion up to now has pointed indirectly to the many problems that confront mental health centers, psychiatrists, and interested citizens as they struggle with the frustratingly complex issues of community mental health. There are two large classes of such problems, one that may be called intrinsic and the other extrinsic. Intrinsic refers to those that primarily stem from the mix of people and programs in a given center in which citizen participation is occurring; extrinsic refers to those of the social, economic, ideological, and political milieu in which the center exists. The practical value of this distinction will hopefully be evident. Since this handbook is intended for a largely professional audience, a problem will mostly be defined as that which is a problem for the professional, although from other viewpoints the professional himself may be a considerable problem. For example, the "average dedicated professional" (to paraphrase Winnicott's excellent term) is usually one who is 5 years or more out of training (meaning that the rapidly emerging citizen participation movement is mostly unfamiliar) and who is trained in a given service discipline (meaning that population-oriented skills are also largely unfamiliar), and whose discipline requires some years of postcollege training (meaning that professional status is important and paraprofessional careers and street-professionals will be mostly unfamiliar). However, these issues belong in a discussion of ''problems citizens have in working with mental health professionals''—which would take us afield.

Problems Intrinsic to the Center

Quality and type of community involvement. These are problems of first importance. As in love or any other social relationship, the quality and type of involvement are fickle, unpredictable, and variable. Confusion might have been less if government regulations had been more specific about the roles and responsibilities of consumers and providers. As Moynihan has noted, the phrase ''maximum feasible participation'' translates easily to ''maximum feasible misunderstanding.''[18] However, it is doubtful that more specific regulations would have helped, due to the power of situational and social forces that come into play when consumers and providers actually sit down together. For example, in some settings, especially rural and suburban areas, the major problem is how to get consumers involved in the first place.

In sharp contrast to this is the ghetto problem of how to handle community involvement. So much felt helplessness and powerlessness have accumulated in the ghetto that many of its residents are not satisfied until they have attained control of every aspect of center policy. They will be satisfied only with levels 7 and 8 in Table 11-3. Control of hiring and firing, signing pay checks, and day-by-day active involvement in the center's administration are inevitable. And, if the center becomes really accepted, it will become a meeting place and a community resource. This sounds fine until one begins to calculate the costs of keeping the center open nights, added secretarial costs, duplicating costs, and so on. Community participation requires large investments of time, money, work, and thought in addition to those required for clinical services. Besides the obvious logistical problems, several less evident ones arise. For example, some center personnel object to having Black Power and La Raza posters and slogans prominantly displayed around the clinic. In many ghetto areas the need for meetings at night means an increased likelihood of being held up and robbed, although this is a daytime problem as well. Finally, and most importantly, very few professionels have the skills and empathy to handle the complicated demands that result from community acceptance and involvement. Some centers have adapted by creating new positions for local residents as community organizers, mental health educators, and the like. This has enabled them to hire people who have the skills and know the community. But unfortunately many centers have not done this, either because of nonrecognition of the need or because of funding problems.

Types of activities and programs associated with community involvement. This is the second major problem area. A good example is the degree to which the use of neighborhood centers is advocated over use of in-hospital care. This not only upsets health professionals, who are most comfortable in a hospital setting, but it means that the center's income is apt to suffer since in-hospital care is much better supported by third-party payers than other types of care.

A related problem is that new approaches to mental health services will be advocated much more rapidly than most professionals can accept comfortably. Specifically the new careers and paraprofessional programs offer the possibility of valued and meaningful work plus credentials without the long and impossible-to-meet requirements of present professional programs. Further, the roles of community liaison, prevention, and advocacy look much more productive as long-run goals than the often frustrating work with difficult people who have already developed mental problems.

Competition for scarce resources and ideological differences.   These will be greatly heightened and complicated by community involvement. This is obvious; however, several less obvious aspects should be mentioned, if only in the hope that anticipatory guidance may help. First, as in any other type of political work, as I believe directing a community mental health center ineluctably is, the point of the game is to win, by fairness when possible. Vince Lombardi is reputed to have said: "Show me a good loser, and I'll show you a loser." A community mental health center director simply cannot afford to lose very often if he wants to remain the director. How he is to accomplish this challenging task is, however, seldom mentioned in training programs—an omission which probably accounts for the exceptionally high job mortality rate of center directors.

Second, most professionals are not apt to undertake such a frontier-type[19] job as working in an urban community mental health center unless they have a very strong commitment toward the view that health and mental health services are human services that should be impartially available—as a right, not a privilege. This is certainly good, meaning I support this view, but it becomes ever more important that center professionals know and can accept the prophetic accuracy of Schuchter's 1968 prediction:

> But the largest segment of the electorate, for the foreseeable future, seems disposed to seek the following goals, probably in this order of priority: maintain racial segregation; reduce crime and social deviance as it impinges upon their safety and comfort; spend less money for welfare objectives benefiting the "undeserving poor," and wipe out slums which impair downtown expansion and renewal.[20]

Added to the need to be a winner, this means that center professionals must also be prepared to exist with humble goals and cultivate available allies to a degree that is mindblowing in relation to the average socialization and training of professionals.

How do you know who is truly representative of the community?   This question has bedeviled and frustrated center directors and everyone else involved in the process of getting more citizen input. There has been a great deal of inexperience, naiveté, and ignorance on the part of many mental health professionals about the nature of this process. Considering the newness and paucity of community-oriented training this is unavoidable, but it has been expensive in terms of time, tempers, and trust. Alinsky, who has had a lifetime of experience with community organizing, has listed the characteristics of a bona fide community organization, of which the following is an abbreviated summary:

> It is this lack of bona fide legitimate community organization which was one of the major rocks on which the Poverty Program foundered. . . . One cannot play charades with this issue and set up stooge committees or reach out for self-appointed, self-annointed, so-called community leaders. . . . What is meant here by bona fide community organization is . . . (1) It is rooted . . . in short, in local people. (2) Its energy . . . is generated by the self-interest of the local residents for the welfare of their children and themselves. (3) Its program for action develops hand in hand with the organization of the community council. . . . (4) It involves a substantial degree of individual citizen participation . . . volunteer activities . . . numerous local committees. . . . (5) It constantly recognizes the functional interrelationship between problems and therefore its program is as broad as the social horizon of the community. It avoids . . . circumscribed and segmental programs. . . . (6) It recognizes that a democratic society is one which responds to popular pressures, and therefore realistically operates on the basis of pressure. For the same reason it does not shy away from involvement in matters of controversy. (7) It concentrates on the utilization of indigenous individuals, who, if not leaders in the beginning, can be developed into leaders. (8) It gives priority to the significance of self-interest. . . . (9) It becomes completely self-financed."[16]

The ways in which community mental health centers have attempted to handle the problem of representativeness are discussed in the final section of this chapter.

Problems Extrinsic to the Center

Real power lies elsewhere.   A number of people have pointed this out, one of the best discussions being by Jonas.[24] He believes that community control is illusory, diversionary, and retrogressive. Illusory, because real control involves control of the essential components of health services. For an institution these are the capital structure, the expense budget, and the staff. For the larger health system (what there is of one), real control involves the patterns of practice, organization, and financing. It is clear that any local community, especially if black and poor, can control none of these essential components. Next, Jonas argues community control is diversionary because it distracts from the real power need for political alliances of patients, community groups, unions, and health workers. Thus, developing political and organizational linkages is more appropriate. Finally, Jonas feels community control is retrogressive because it pits powerless consumers against powerless providers, a struggle which can only cause further deterioration of care.

Opposed to this view are those who argue that those involved in control of the essential institutional and system components are neither monolithic nor unsympathetic to the problems and the need for change. For example, it is hard to conceive that an institution or system can for long remain consciously ineffective, racist, or aloof from community needs. The last 5–10 years have made it steadily more difficult for health institutions and others to avoid being conscious of these defects. Thus there has been a wide variety of intended correctives in many areas of health services, which appear to be so useful they warrant wider application. A few examples are the Joint Commission on Accreditation of Hospitals, a "bill of rights" for patients, the hiring of patient advocates, and the enlarged role of consumers on hospital, regional, national, and third-party boards and committees. Some feel that consumerism is simply another fad and will be out in a few years. However, given the rising costs and public interest, it seems reasonable to believe that consumerism and community involvement will continue to grow and expand until some form of national health insurance is enacted, at which point the pattern may change drastically. Even so, it is difficult to imagine that such legislation and its implementation will be unaffected by the citizen and community movement. In fact, it may well be that national health legislation will greatly expand the role of nonmedical and nonprofessional parties in all levels of policy making.

Mental health care is a new health service and its scope remains poorly defined. This has a number of implications for policymaking. In addition to the ideological differences mentioned earlier, there are enormous and presently insoluble ambiguities in the field that we simply have to live with. Returning to the example of surgical appendectomy compared to mental disorder. If treatment of a straightforward condition like appendicitis is so profoundly influenced by the characteristics of the health service system, how much more must the mental health field be influenced? One could, without too much stretching, even make a case for the idea that the more mental health professionals there are, the more mental health cases there must be, i.e., professionals "cause" mental illness by putting a label on emotional upset. The recent report of normal people who got themselves hospitalized and their "disorder" diagnosed as "schizophrenia in remission"[22] is simply one especially telling instance of this. Much wider appreciation of labeling and the various hidden conceptual models in mental health and psychiatry, as in an excellent recent paper by Lazare[23], is needed if the field is to achieve some reliability and validity.

This is important to policymaking for two major reasons: (1) the bewilderment of community advisory groups in trying to learn what the issues are, and (2) the reluctance of legislators to support something about which everyone is so divided. If, as Lazare suggests, we can agree that "human beings are simultaneously biologic organisms, psychologic selves, behaving animals, and members of social systems," and that no profession has the answers, it should be easier for neuropsychiatrists, psychoanalysts, behaviorists, and community mental healthers to agree that each is looking at a different part of the elephant called "human beings in distress." In turn, our public image might be much more coherent and our policy problems a bit more manageable.

Most apparent causes of mental disorder remain beyond anyone's control. We do not yet have the proved ability to prevent mental disorder, as for example we do poliomyelitis and many infectious diseases. There are certainly many promising developments[24] but the field is still in an early phase. Despite this my experience has been that citizen board members are much more convinced of the worth of preventively oriented programs than professionals are. This means that professionals need to get better acquainted with preventive and public health psychiatry if they are to be useful in decisionmaking.

In addition, what we do know about the prevention of mental disorders suggests that socioeconomic and environmental stresses are extremely important factors. This in turn implies that effective interventions must involve other social institutions. Although this means that the influence of the mental health professions is further limited, it also means that the support of a knowledgeable and concerned community can be of immeasurable help. For example, a legislator will listen far more attentively to citizens' groups seeking support for mental health programs than he will to psychiatrists seeking the same.

WHAT ARE SOME SOLUTIONS?

This section concerns itself solely with the levels of citizen participation listed in Table 11-3 that involve genuine citizen power: partnership, delegated power, and citizen control. Since in all three some degree of partnership is involved, ramifications of this will be discussed first.

Partnership is defined in the *Oxford Universal Dictionary* as "an association of two or more persons for the carrying on of a business, of which they share the expenses, profit and loss." In our specific case it means sharing in the problems and responsibilities of running a community mental health center that have been discussed earlier. The most straightforward partnership arrangement is that of a private, incorporated, nonprofit mental health center. In this case a group of citizens and professionals concerned about meeting mental health needs bands together and creates an organization. As a corporate body these people can seek funding from the community and other sources such as the state or federal government and third-party payers. A number of hospitals and child guidance clinics have found this a practical structure, and some community mental health centers have followed the pattern. The oldest of these to my knowledge is the Wellesley Human Relations Service established in 1953 in Massachusetts. In these corporate mental health organizations, policy is made by a board of directors and implemented by the staff. A psychiatrist is usually the executive director, but not always. Appointment of new members to the board, designation of term of office, etc., are controlled by the board according to its particular bylaws.

Unfortunately, this logical and simple organizational model is not possible in many situations, especially in the large cities. The degree of public government control makes it difficult or impossible to use a private sector model. For example, in many states all the community mental health centers are based in state-run mental hospitals or clinics. In other cases the size, importance, and quasi-public nature of the large urban hospitals makes it difficult to add new (e.g., poor, minority) citizens to their policy process. Yet another major difference is the unequal status of the prospective partners. For a partnership even to exist, each partner must bring something sufficiently valuable to make his association desirable. For example, until recent past years it was not understood what a black minister or a welfare mother might contribute to a board of directors when compared, say, with a banker. This aspect of the partnership quid pro quo has undergone rapid change in the health and human services for the reasons mentioned earlier: Citizen participation may bring correctives to ineffective or irrelevant service (consumers are experts in the mistakes of medical services), to institutionalized racist or other exclusionary practices, and to the dangers of destruction and violence toward buildings and personnel. In short, it has been recognized that citizens/consumers/residents in the large city ghettos bring a great deal to a health service partnership.

The next issue then is *which* citizens bring these resources? How does a mental health center find out who has the interest, knowledge, and influence to enter into a partnership relationship with the center to promote common goals? The solution suggested by Alinsky earlier is certainly an excellent one, namely, to attach mental health services to an existing community organization, as is the case with the Woodlawn Organization in Chicago. However, this is not always possible, so the problem remains. The following are published examples of various attempts at solution.

Martin Luther King Jr. Health Center

This center in the Bronx has attempted to get community policy input by holding an annual election. Anyone wishing to serve on the board is required to get 25 signatures on a petition. In the year described, 52 people did this, and 21 of them became members of the center's policy board. It was noted that this was a very small sample of the 45,000-person community, less than 1000 signatures or 2 percent of the population.[25] This lack of community response has been noted in other government projects and undoubtedly has to do with the unwillingness of urban residents to get involved in anything unless its relevance and self-interest are clear. On the other hand, given time and a great deal of promotional work, it is possible to get a much better turnout. For example, the Columbia Point (Boston) Health Association elections are said to turn out about 40 percent of eligible voters.

Health Center in Watts (Los Angeles)

The 25-member board of this center contains 17 members from the area and 6 members from outside. The 6 outside members are selected on the basis of needed expertise (medicine, law, finance, business, etc.), while the 17 resident members are selected on the basis of equal parts of chance and demographical representativeness. Each census tract is represented by one to two members, depending on the size of the tract, and the overall composition of the residents is intended to mirror the adult community characteristics of age, sex, and ethnicity. When a vacancy occurs or a term expires, the center advertises for nominees who fit these characteristics. All nominees' names are put in a hat and the person's

name withdrawn is offered a place on the board. This process is certainly fair
enough, but it does not necessarily attract people who can participate effectively.
Both this center and the one in the Bronx attempt to correct this problem by providing training for board members. Indeed training is a key element in all centers
attempting to develop genuine community involvement. Two rather provocative
statements describe it thus:

> It may be that the poor are never "ready" to assume power in an advanced society:
> the exercise of power in an effective manner is an ability acquired through apprenticeship
> and seasoning. Thrust on an individual or group, the results are often painful to observe,
> and when what in fact is conveyed is not power, but a kind of playacting at power, the
> results can be absurd.[18]

> There is a legitimate concern that the poor will continue to receive second class health
> care, only this time delivered by their neighbors instead of by professionals from outside
> their community. . . . Some feel that the control exercised by their board ought to weed
> out these employees who do not meet quality standards, but that, in reality, many boards
> use their power to make firing a rare action indeed. . . . What does this do to patient
> care?[26]

These comments point to the need for training in how to be a board member
for the new citizen/consumer participants. This is undoubtedly valuable as a partial or temporary solution, and those who have been involved in the community
board training programs have generally found them of great value. There is also
a need for professional/provider training, as has been indicated earlier in the
comments on the "unfit fitness" of psychiatrists. Little has been written on this,
although Galiher has made a few suggestions,[27] and I have recommended that
local psychiatric associations donate volunteer time to ghetto mental health centers
in order to acquire some insight and sensitivity to the problems.

The Westside Community Mental Health Center, Inc.

This example in my experience represents an effective policy structure, although its applicability to other areas is obviously unknown. This is the experimental consortium or partnership of some 15 mental health agencies and the community area designated as the Westside area of San Francisco. The center itself
has been described in a number of other writings[28,29] so the focus here is restricted
to policymaking and community involvement.

The major characteristic of the policy apparatus is its double-board structure,
a policy board and a community board. In the development of the center it was
recognized that both the service structure and the community structure were too
complex to permit adequate representation of those who needed to have a voice
in making decisions. For example, the community contained a large black ghetto
(Western Addition—Filmore), the Haight-Ashbury district, Japantown, a presti-
gious white area (Pacific Height–Marina), and many transitional areas. Similarly
the service structure included a number of major hospitals, family social service

agencies, halfway houses, drug-treatment programs, and other specialized mental health organizations.

In addition to the variety there were vast discrepancies in interest, aims, knowledge, service capacity, and funding among the many participants. The double-board structure was therefore created to give this complex mixture enough form and regularity to enable delivery of mental health services. The community advisory board served to represent as many of the diverse interests of the community as possible. Membership on the community advisory board came by way of an annual, well-publicized community forum at which the center reports on its activities and open discussion and elections are held. Especially in the beginning it was necessary for the originators to spend careful thought and long hours in identifying and contacting representative and influential individuals and community organizations in order to win their agreement to participate in the center. Fortunately for the center, San Francisco had undergone a series of long and violent battles over urban renewal with the result that indigenous community organization was quite advanced, and indigenous leadership was sophisticated in the detection of token participation. Thus, once this leadership decided that the center was possibly sincere in wanting citizen input, good turnout and capable and influential community representation were not difficult to obtain. This community advisory board had the following functions: (1) to assist in meeting the needs of area residents, (2) to serve as the conscience of the community, (3) to help in letting the community know of the availability of services, (4) to aid in improving coordination of care, (5) to elect members who will constitute 50 percent of the board of directors.

Functions 2 and 5 are the major avenues for policy input from the community. Because they have different implications for citizen participation in community mental health, they merit brief discussion.

The conscience of the community. Although this is a high-sounding phrase that could easily become shallow rhetoric, my experience has been that people generally take it seriously. Many people, whether poor people or professional people, know that there are serious defects in human service programs. The problem is how to get together constructively. Thus, an articulate and representative community advisory board can be an excellent mechanism. Take the following example in which the community advisory board was essential. Since this is published elsewhere,[9] I focus only on the policy aspects. A 5-year-old black girl was kicked by a chronically psychotic white male, resulting in bleeding and distress on the part of both the child and her mother. Although the mother sought the usual medical and legal help, she was turned away. A black militant self-help group learned of the mother's plight and brought it to the attention of the Westside staff and the community advisory board. The staff's reaction was mixed. Everyone was sorry the incident had happened, but what needed to be done was less clear. Some were outraged and indignant, while others felt that the refusal of medical help by the hospital was a "regrettable breakdown in communication" between a black ghetto mother and a middle-class white nurse. In any case the staff's reaction was sufficiently varied that no clear response would have emerged. Certainly the staff would not have wholeheartedly supported the militant neighborhood group's threats to bomb or set fire to the hospital. In contrast, the reaction of the community advisory board was one of uniform outrage. It pointed out that (1) chronically psychotic white patients should not be placed in the ghetto in the first place (the man was in a state-supported board-and-care home); he should be cared for in a white neighborhood where such incidents would be less inflammatory; (2) the hospital should not have nurses in the emergency room who are unable to understand neighborhood residents, as it is simply too dangerous in urgent matters involving life and death; (3) it could appreciate the militant group's thesis that a violent response was called for. The hospital's refusal to apologize and transfer the nurse to a less sensitive position was yet another instance of institutional callousness that only seemed to change when violence was threatened. As a result of the clarity of the community response, the center's staff received some needed education about the facts of life in the ghetto and the center was able to respond unambiguously. Examples similar to this are legion in community mental health work and make this "conscience function" an extremely important input to center policy making.

Election of 50 of the board of directors. This function of the community advisory board helps assure that the community sends its best people to represent it on the board level. For example, those who already hold respected positions of power in the community tend to be elected. Conversely, community members who don't attend the meetings regularly or who don't grasp the issues are not apt to be elected. Thus, the community half of the board of directors tends to be knowledgeable, articulate, and hardworking. The result is that the community members are well able to deal with the institutional members on an equal basis, are able to relate as true partners. This does not mean that everyone gets along smoothly. It does mean that the fights are more apt to be equal and the resulting outcomes more apt to be better compromises.

A Mental Health Center Which Has Used Delegated Power

This type of community participation refers to cases in which the community mental health center delegates authority and responsibility for a portion of its program to a community organization that has special expertise or qualifications. In effect, the center subcontracts for a part of its needs. Although this is a well-established mechanism in business, it has seldom been used in the mental health field. The center that has probably had the most experience with this is the Community Mental Health Center at the University of Illinois Medical Center Complex. The director of the center, Dr. Harvey Freed, has recently described his impressions of their 2-year experience with subcontracting for mental health services in the black community.[30,31] This interesting development came about as the result of complementary needs in both the center and the community, although this was not recognized initially. From the standpoint of the center, community development was an important goal, hence the staff made efforts to develop community advisory groups. From the standpoint of the militant black community, the medical center and its programs were suspect as being Establishment, racist, and irrelevant. The community was more interested in confrontation and taking over than entering into a useless discussion. After a number of unsatisfactory attempts to get community involvement, Freed took the courageous and creative step of letting two of the militant groups operate their own programs. Although 2 years is a short time to evaluate the outcome, it certainly appears that both the center and the militant community have moved from a highly polarized relationship to one where there are increasing areas of agreement. Thus, in settings where polarization or other forces work against partnership relationships, this type of delegated control may be a useful method. Although Freed doesn't emphasize it, it is important to note that simply delegating authority for conducting some type of program doesn't solve the problem. Running any type of service program in the ghetto requires much more than community support and program relevance. The needs for administrative support, fiscal expertise, familiarity with local, state, and federal regulations are gigantic. Thus, the center can be extremely helpful in sharing what expertise it has in these matters with the community organization it has subcontracted or delegated to. Ironically, centers themselves tend to be deficient in staffing for such managerial functions, so this sharing is easier said than done at present. However, if community mental health centers survive the current Nixon administration assault on social programs (I predict those with strong community support will), managerial support must develop and hopefully be available as a significant contribution to the community development regarding mental health services.

CONCLUDING REMARKS

We have covered an enormous range of subject matter since asking the deceptively simple question, Who decides what happens in a community mental health center? Undoubtedly other writers would stress other aspects, especially in a more systematic discussion of policy. My aim, in keeping with that of a practitioner-oriented handbook, has been to select those aspects that most center directors and staff will encounter. However, readers should be alerted to the fact that community mental health policy is a subcategory of social policy, especially as it relates to the public sector. Social policy in turn is a very broad area about which a great deal has been written. Thus, those with special interest in community mental health policy should review that literature. Similarly, policy making in community mental health *centers* is a subcategory of the larger areas of organizations, administration, and management, and there is much to be learned there.

Bearing all the above limitations in mind, this chapter has attempted to select the following emphases as relevant to community mental health center policy:

1. The ghetto community mental health center is the most interesting psychiatric institution that presently exists. The mental health professions, especially psy-

chiatry, have an unparalleled opportunity to innovate in both service patterns and administrative patterns.

2. Citizen involvement in mental health policy making is almost certain to increase, especially with regard to consumers and neighborhood residents of low income and minority ethnic status.

3. This involvement creates both problems and opportunities. The problems include much additional time and expense and unaccustomed sharing of power and responsibility among groups that have wide sociological differences. Unpleasant conflict will be frequent, and issues such as racism and ideological differences along the mental health–mental illness continuum will be omnipresent.

4. The opportunities include strengthening the community sanction and political support for mental health and improving the range and fit of mental health professionals and programs.

5. It is important to keep in mind that the scope of decisionmaking has changed radically with the shift to community mental health centers. The crucial decisions are no longer treatment decisions, but rather are decisions involving money, community relations, power, and deployment of scarce resources.

6. Finally, the role of psychiatrists in this decisional process is complex and still being defined. The complexity stems from the conflict of interest resulting from the scarcity of psychiatric resources and the differing orientations among psychiatrists. The lack of definition is simply a reflection of the fact that a major sociopolitical change has occurred in mental health in the recent past. In following this development, the ghetto mental health center may be considered as the leading edge or indicator of the forces involved.

REFERENCES

1. American Psychiatric Association: Position statement on community mental health centers. Am J Psychiatry 130:239–240, 1973

2. Mechanic D: Mental Health and Social Policy. Englewood Cliffs, NJ, Prentice-Hall, 1969

3. Joint Commission on Mental Illness and Health. Action for Mental Health. New York, Basic Books, 1961.

4. Howe L: The concept of the community: Some implications for the development of community psychiatry. In Bellak L (ed): Handbook of Community Psychiatry and Community Mental Health. New York, Grune & Stratton, 1964.

5. Wilder JF, Levin G, Zwerling I: Planning and developing the locus of care. In Grunebaum H (ed): The Practice of Community Mental Health. Boston, Little, Brown, 1970

6. Panzetta AF: Community Mental Health: Myth and Reality. Philadelphia, Lea & Febiger, 1971

7. Roman M, Schmais A: Consumer participation and control: A conceptual overview. In Barten HH, Bellak L (eds): Progress in Community Mental Health, vol II. New York, Grune & Stratton, 1972

8. Bolman WM: Community control of the community mental health center. I. Introduction. Am J Psychiatry 129:173–180, 1972

9. Bolman WM: Community control of the community mental health center. II. Case examples. Am J Psychiatry 129:181–186, 1972

10. Lewis CE: Variations in the incidence of surgery. N Engl J Med 281:880–884, 1969

11. Leopold RL: Urban problems and the community mental health center: Multiple mandates, difficult choices. Am J Orthopsychiatry 41:144–167, 1971

12. Whittington HG: In Glasscote RM, Sussex JN, Cumming E, Smith LH (eds): The Community Mental Health Center: An Interim Appraisal. Washington DC, Joint Information Service, 1969

13. Center for Minority Group Mental Health Programs, National Institute of Mental Health: Bibliography on Racism. Washington DC, GPO, 1972

14. Thomas A, Sillen S: Racism and Psychiatry. New York, Brunner/Mazel, 1972

15. Arnstein SR: A ladder of citizen participation. Am Inst Planners J 35:216–224, 1969

16. Alinsky, SD: What is the role of community organization in bargaining with the establishment for health care services? In Norman J C (ed): Medicine in the Ghetto. New York, Appleton, 1969

17. American Medical Association Committee on Health Care of the Poor: Cited in Med World News, May 19, 1972, pp 51–63

18. Moynihan D L: Maximum Feasible Misunderstanding. New York, Free Press (Macmillan) 1969

19. Abrams C: The City Is the Frontier. New York, Harper & Row, 1965

20. Schuchter A: White Power/Black Freedom. Boston, Beacon Press, 1968

21. Jonas S: A theoretical approach to the question of "community control" of health service facilities. Am J Public Health 61:916–921, 1971

22. Rosenhan DL: On being sane in insane places. Science 179:250–258, 1973

23. Lazare A: Hidden conceptual models in clinical psychiatry. New Engl J Med 288:345–351, 1973

24. Bolman WM: Toward realizing the prevention of mental illness. In Bellak L, Barten HH (eds): Progress in Community Mental Health, vol I. New York, Grune & Stratton, 1969

25. Peck RL: Community control: The real struggle begins. Hosp Physician 5:57–59, 139–143, 1971

26. Editorial: What price community control? Community Health Forum, vol 1, no 4, New York, New Careers Training Laboratory, New York University, 1971

27. Galiher CB, Needleman J, Rolfe CJ: Consumer participation. HMSA Health Rep 86:99–106, 1971

28. Bolman WM, Goldman W: The San Francisco Westside Community Mental Health Center, Inc.: Development of a mental health consortium of private agencies. In Levenson AI, Beigel A (eds): The Community Mental Health Center: Strategies and Programs. New York, Basic Books, 1972

29. Bolman WM: The mental health consortium. In Barten HH, Bellak, L (eds): Progress in Community Mental Health, vol II. New York, Grune & Stratton, 1972

30. Freed HM: Promoting accountability in mental health services: The negotiated mandate. Am J Orthopsychiatry 42:761–770, 1972

31. Freed HM: Subcontracts for community development and service. Am J Psychiat 129:568–573, 1972

Index

Accountability
  challenge of, 207–209
  obligation for, 216
Action for Mental Health, 220
Activity group therapy, 22
Addiction, 1
  see also Drug abuse
Adolescence, drug abuse and, 141–142
Advertising, drug abuse and, 144–145
Aged
  day-care program for, 94
  in French district psychiatry, 82–83
  mental health services for, 91–93
  psychiatric needs of, 91–103
  psychopathology and depression in, 92
  see also Old age
Albert Einstein College of Medicine, 18
Alcohol
  ambivalent attitude toward, 163
  drugs and, 168–169, 176
Alcoholic(s)
  criminal prosecution of, 165
  defined, 165
  dependence in, 131
  at Guidance Center of New Rochelle, 66
  loss of control in, 166
  number of in U.S., 163
  problems and troubles of, 166
  self-destructive attitude in, 166

  treatment for, 173–177
Alcoholics Anonymous, 165, 177
Alcoholism, 1, 163–178
  Antabuse and, 176
  aversion therapy in, 176
  community program and, 172–174
  confidentiality in, 172
  defined, 168
  destructive behavior in, 175
  detoxification in, 174–177
  diagnosis of, 169–171
  as disease, 163, 174
  disulfiram (Antabuse) in, 176
  drugs and, 168–169, 176
  drunken driving and, 170
  early detection of, 169–172
  epidemic of, 167
  family and, 177
  father-son relationship in, 171
  follow-up and evaluation in, 177–178
  at Guidance Center of New Rochelle, 63
  group therapy in, 177
  history of, 163–165
  individual treatment in, 166
  lithium carbonate in, 176
  medical profession and, 169
  prevention and education in, 167–169
  related offenses and, 165
  society and, 177

stigma of, 164–165
symptoms of, 170
women and, 171
tranquilizers and, 168, 176
treatment in, 166, 174–177
WHO definition of, 165
Allied Services Act (1972), 198
American Hospital Association, 169
American Medical Association, 229
American Psychiatric Association, 4, 15, 219–220
Amitriptyline, in psychotic depression, 20
Antabuse (disulfiram), 176
Antagonist maintenance program, in drug abuse, 153–155
Antidrug peer culture, 142–143
Antipsychiatry, 4
Antipsychotic drugs, 16
Art therapy, 22
Asch, S. E., 212
Association of Mental Health (Paris), 69 n., 71–73

Bazelon, Judge, 102–103
Baltimore, children's services in, 107–108
Barbiturates, alcohol and, 168 see also Drug(s)
Barten, Harvey, 43–67
Behavior modification, 21
Bellak, Leopold, 1–11, 215
Bendit, E. A., 175
Berlin, Irving N., 105–123
Berman, M., 7
Black children, counseling and therapeutic services for, 53–54
Black ghetto, in Westside (San Francisco) area, 235–236, 239–240
Black Muslims, 158
Black psychiatrists, in Guidance Center of New Rochelle, 54
Black psychologists, 54
Bloom, B. S., 210
Blue Cross Association, 31
Bolman, William M., 188, 219–240
Boulding, K. E., 194
Brody, Stanley J., 198 n.
Bronx-Lebanon Hospital, 28
Bronx Municipal Hospital Center, 20

Bronx State Hospital, 9
general description of, 18–19
hotel ward at, 24
liaison programs at, 25–29
multimodality approach in, 22–23
occupational therapy at, 22
residential programs of, 23–25
supportive therapy at, 20–21
therapeutic community approach in, 21
treatment programs at, 19–23
Westside Center and, 36–40
Bunyan, Paul, 164

California
community programs in, 93
Medicaid program in, 35
number of mental patients in, 17
California Department of Mental Hygiene, 32
California Medical Clinic for Psychotherapy, 32
Campbell, D. T., 215–216
Catchment area concept, 186
Center for the Study of Responsive Law, 37
Chafetz, Morris E., 163–178
Charcot, Jean Martin, 71
Chicago, Woodlawn community mental health centers in, 106
Child development, education of professionals in, 114
Childhood
crisis intervention and comprehensive care in, 114–115
developmentally based mental health activities for, 110–119
health-mental health model in, 109
learning and skills acquisition in, 116–118
maternal depression and, 110–112
mental health activity in, 116–118
mental health consultation for, 118–119
multipurpose approach in, 109
preschool preventive mental health and, 112–113
school as mental health resource in, 115–116
supportive networks and, 122
Childhood psychiatry, 105–123

Children
    counseling services for, 51–52
    crisis intervention for, 113–115, 119–120
    day hospital care for, 121
    evaluation of services for, 123
    group homes and foster homes for,
        121–122
    inpatient care for, 121
    mental health centers for, 118
    mental health consultation for, 118–119
    outpatient services for, 121
    special education for, 118
    team approach to services for, 122
    therapeutic schools and day-care centers
        for, 120
    see also Childhood; Children's mental
        health services
Children's mental health services
    at Guidance Center of New Rochelle,
        51–53
    models of, 106–107
    paraprofessionals in, 106, 109, 114
    spectrum of, 119–122
Chlordiazepoxide, alcohol and, 168
Chlorpromazine, 10
    alcoholism and, 168
Citizen participation
    ideology in, 224–225
    jobs and, 227
    persons and interests in, 223
    policy aspects of, 219–240
    racism and, 227
    type of involvement in, 227–229
CHMC, see Community mental health
    center
Columbia Point (Boston) Health
    Association, 235
Community
    conscience of, 237
    drug use and, 134–138
Community Chest funds, 35
Community involvement, 188
    activities and programs associated with,
        230–231
    in general health care, 198–199
    ideology and, 231
    see also Citizen participation
Community mental health

accountability in, 207–209
clinical intervention and community
    response in, 206–207
contemporary scene in, 10–11
future directions of, 9
heroic stage in, 2
niche breadth and exploratory behavior in,
    211–212
nonmedical model for, 205–216
overview of, 1–11
turnover of system linkage in, 212–216
Community mental health center
    backward look at, 183–192
    catchment area concept in, 186
    children in, 105–123
    chronically psychotic patient in, 17
    citizen participation in, 219–240
    community representatives in, 231–232
    complementarity of systems in, 119–202
    consultation and education in, 189–190
    continuing education and esprit in, 59–60
    crisis intervention in, 114–115
    delegated power in, 238–239
    developmentally based, 110–119
    drug abuse and, 142
    elderly in, 98–100
    emerging problems of, 56–67
    establishment of, 3
    evaluation of, 185–192
    external problems and, 232–234
    fiscal problems of, 61–65
    funding problems of, 183–185, 226–227
    ghetto and, 235–236, 239–240
    ideologies and, 231
    jobs in, 227
    liaison with hospital, 26
    mental retardation programs in, 190–191
    paraprofessional aides in, 59
    partnership in, 234
    patient flow in, 16
    prevention syndrome in, 187
    primary focus of, 16
    priorities in, 225–226
    problems of, 229–234
    solutions to problems in, 234–239
    staffing of, 57–58
    strengths and weaknesses of, 186
    suburban setting for, 45–46

training and, 201–202
training for elderly in, 101
two-class care system in, 191
at University of Illinois, 238–239
Community Mental Health Centers Act
    (1963), 2, 11, 43–67, 189, 220
Community mental health services, old age
    and, 98
Community psychiatry
    artifacts of, 8–9
    vs. district psychiatry, 74, 80–81
    drug therapy and, 5
    evolution in, 2
    in heroic phase, 3
    in Paris, 69–87
    psychosis and, 5–8
    third revolution in, 2
    see also Community mental health
Community resources centers, drug abuse
    and, 147–148
Community response, clinical intervention
    and, 206–207
Compazine, 168
Comprehensive Alcohol Abuse and
    Alcoholism Prevention Treatment and
    Rehabilitation Act (1970), 165
Comprehensive Health Center, liaison with
    mental hospital, 27–28
Conrad House, 32
"Consumer," poor as, 33
Creative arts therapies, 22–23
Crime, drug use and, 135
Crisis intervention, in childhood mental
    illness, 114–115, 119–120
Crotona Park mental health service, 27–28

Dance therapy, 22
Day care
    for children, 121
    for elderly, 94
Day hospital program, 24
    at Guidance Center of New Rochelle,
        49–51
Daytop, drug abuse and, 139, 558
Denone, H. W., Jr., 166
Depersonalization, 5
Depression, age and, 92
Detoxification

alcoholism and, 174
drug abuse and, 155
Deutsch, M., 213
developmental tasks, mental illness and,
    210–211
Disease
    alcoholism as, 163, 174
    drug use and, 132
District psychiatry
    aged and, 82–83
    care of families in, 83–85
    child and adult departments in, 75
    vs. community psychiatry, 80–81
    continuity of care in, 75–82
    development and organization of, 72
    professional principles in, 74–75
    research and teaching in, 85–86
    responsibility in, 75–82
    in 13th arrondissement, Paris, 71–86
Disturbed children, 105–123
    see also Childhood; children
Disulfiram (Antabuse), 176
Dole, V. P., 56
Drinking behavior, 170
    see also Alcoholic(s); Alcoholism
Driver decision, 165
Drug(s)
    alcoholism and, 176
    availability of, 132
    defined, 130
    dependence on, 131
    experimental or recreational use of, 130
    illegal, 130
    social factors in, 132
    socioeconomic factors in, 132
Drug abuse, 129–161
    in adolescence, 141–142
    advertising and, 144–145
    alpha wave conditioning in, 160
    antidrug peer culture and, 142–143
    behavioral conditioning in, 159
    carbon dioxide inhalation therapy in, 159
    cause of, 131–132
    community resources centers and,
        147–148
    community response to, 136–138
    criminal behavior and, 135
    definitions in, 130–131
    detoxification in, 155

drug education and, 138–141, 148
ex-addict's role in prevention of, 139
experimental approaches in treatment of, 159–160
group approach in prevention of, 142
group homes and, 148–149
group therapy in, 155–156
hepatitis and, 141
heroin maintenance in, 153
individual aid in, 147–149
LSD therapy in, 159–160
maintenance in, 151–154
mass media and, 144–145
mental health programs and, 144
methadone maintenance in, 152
narcotic antagonists in, 153–155
outreach and treatment in, 149–150
primary prevention in, 138–146
recreational facilities and, 147–148
religion-oriented programs and, 157–159
secondary prevention in, 146–150
self-help residential therapeutic communities in, 155–156
socioeconomic conditions and, 143
tacit community support of, 149
tertiary prevention in, 150–160
traditional psychotherapy in, 156
Drug-abuse programs, at Guidance Center of New Rochelle, 55–56
Drug dependence, defined, 131
Drug education, 138–141
Drug laws, 145–146
Drug use
    alternatives to, 143–144
    community influence in, 133–136
    community support of, 149
    defined, 130
    disease and, 132
    drop-in centers for, 157
    see also Drug abuse
Drunken driving, 170
    see also Alcoholism
Duffy, J., 209

Easter decision, 165
Education, drug abuse and, 138–141, 148
Ego functions
    schizophrenia and, 5
    strengthening of, 21

Elderly
    mental health care for, 92–93
    negative attitudes toward, 96
    see also Aged; Old age
Electric convulsive therapy, 10, 19–20
Environment, turnover and system breakage in, 212–216
Erikson, Erik, 210

Family
    abandonment by, 24
    in French district psychiatry, 83–85
    of schizophrenics, 6, 7 n.
Family Service of San Francisco, 32
Feffer, M., 212
Foster homes, 25
France, district psychiatry in, 70–87
Freed, Harvey, 238–239
Freud, Sigmund, 10, 71, 210

General health care, merger with mental health care, 192–202
Geriatrics, negative attitudes toward, 96
Gesell, Arnold, 210
Ghetto community mental health center, 235–236, 239–240
Glidewell, John C., 205–216
Goffman, E., 7
Goldfarb, A. K., 97
Goldman, W., 31–40
Grinspoon, L., 20
Group for the Advancement of Psychiatry, 91, 94, 103
Group homes, drug abuse and, 148–149
Group psychotherapy, at Guidance Center of New Rochelle, 48–49
Group therapy, in drug abuse, 155–156
Guidance Center of New Rochelle
    alcoholics at, 63, 66
    children's counseling services at, 51–53
    children's services at, 51–53
    cost of treatment at, 65
    drug-abuse programs at, 55–56
    "emotional containments" and, 66
    future planning for, 65–67
    group psychotherapy at, 48–49
    limited resources of, 46–47
    location of, 43–44

operation of, 44–46
psychiatric population explosion and, 46
rehabilitation and day hospital programs
   at, 49–51
satellite programs at, 53–55
short-time psychotherapy at, 47–48
therapeutic nursery school at, 53

Haight-Asbury hippie community, 33
Haire, M., 213
Halfway houses, 25
Hallucinations, 5
Hammerson, Marion W., 7 n.
Hand, J., 96
Harrison Act (1914), 145–146
Hauser, P. M., 208, 212
H. Douglas Singer Zone Center, 167
Health, Education and Welfare Department,
   U.S., 9
Health care
   community involvement in, 198–199
   consumer involvement in, 194–195
   similarity of problems in relation to those
      of mental health, 196
   single-payment financing in, 196
Health Insurance Plan of New York City,
   195
Health maintenance organization, 183–202
   Bronx State Hospital and, 27
   compensation in, 195–196
Health mobilization organization, 1
Hepatitis, drug abuse and, 141
Heroin, availability of, 132
Hertzmann, M., 175
"Hertzman" in text; see refs. p. 179
Hoenig, Julius, 7 n.
Hotel ward, at Bronx State Hospital, 24
Howe, L., 221
Hugo, Victor, 71
Human development, illness and, 209
Hunt, J. McV., 210
Hypoproteinemia, 22

Illinois, University of, 238
Illness, human development and, 209
Illness-health continuum, in mental health
   field, 224
Imipramine, in psychotic depression, 20

Insulin shock treatment, 10

Jesus Movement (Jesus Freaks), 158
Jewish Family Service, 32
Joint Commission on Mental Illness and
   Health, 220

Kaiser-Permanente groups, 195
Kasl, S. V., 96
Katz, E., 214
Katzenstein, Rhoda, 69 n.
Kelly, J. G., 211
Kennedy, John F., 2
Kennedy centers, for retarded, 118
Kleber, Herbert D., 129–161
Kohlberg, L., 210
Kuhn, Dorothy S., 183 n.

Lake v. Cameron, 102
Landau, R., 7
Lazarsfeld, P., 214
League School for psychotic children, 118
Learning in childhood, 116–118
Lebovici, Serge, 69–87
Leighton, D., 118
Leopold, Robert L., 183–202
Les Miserables (Hugo), 71
Lewin, K., 215
Liaison programs, Bronx State Hospital,
   25–29
Librium, alcohol and, 168
Lincoln Hospital, 28
Lincoln Hospital Community Mental Health
   Center, 27
Lithium carbonate, alcoholism and, 176
Loomis, C. P., 208, 213
Lowenthal, M. F., 97
LSD (lysergic acid diethylamide), 10, 140
   consciousness change through, 129
   in drug abuse therapy, 159–160

Mansfield, E., 213
Markson, E. W., 96
Martin Luther King Jr. Comprehensive
   Neighborhood Health Center, 27–28,
   235
Massachusetts General Hospital, 167
Mass communication, as system linkage,
   213

Mass media, drug abuse and, 144–145
Maternal depression, 110–112
May, P., 20
Mechanic, David, 220
Medical practice, changes in, 193–194
Medi-Cal program, 35
Medicare-Medicaid reimbursements,
    1967–69, 94–95
Mental health
    community, see Community mental
        health
    consumer involvement in, 194–195
    see also Psychiatry
Mental Health Administration, 198
Mental health care
    defining of, 233
    merger with general health care, 192–202
Mental health care delivery, models for
    organizing of, 31–40
Mental health consultation, 189
Mental health field
    conservative-liberal-radical continuum in,
        224
    health-illness ideologies in, 224–225
    illness-health continuum in, 224
    priority conflict in, 225–226
Mental health movement, "illnesses" in,
    209
Mental health pollution, 8
Mental health services, aging and, 91–92
Mental hospital
    liaison with community mental health
        center, 26–27
    outmoded features of, 15
    unitized, 17
Mental illness
    development tasks and, 210–211
    disequilibrium in, 22
    relatedness in, 21
    role of work in prevention of, 118
    sociopathy in, 21–22
    welfare system and, 191
    see also Mental health field
Mentally ill, laws governing, 4
Mental Retardation Act (1964), 220
Mental retardation programs, 190–191
Meprobamate, alcohol and, 168
Merton, R. K., 215

Methadone maintenance clinics, 44, 56
Metrazol, 19
Milieu therapy, 21
Miller, S. M., 214
Miltown, 168
Moore, W. E., 25
Mt. Zion Hospital, 32, 34
Murphy, G. E., 175
Music therapy, 22

Nader report, 37
Narcotic antagonists, in drug abuse,
    153–155
    see also Drug(s); Drug abuse
Nation, Carrie, 164
National Association for Mental Health,
    219
National Coordinating Council on Drug
    Education, 139–140
National Council on Alcoholism, 170, 172
National Institute on Alcohol Abuse and
    Alcoholism, 163–164, 169, 172
National Institute of Mental Health, 8, 49,
    62–63, 92, 139, 187
National Institutes of Health, 62
National Mental Health Act, 93
New Rochelle, Guidance Center of, see
    Guidance Center of New Rochelle
New York Civil Liberties Union, 4
New York State, number of mental patients
    in, 17
New York State Department of Mental
    Hygiene, 44–45, 49, 61
New York State Narcotics Addiction
    Control Commission, 55, 63
New York Times, 4, 8
Nixon, Richard M., 198
"Noble savage" concept, 6
Noll, Ann, 178
Nursery school, therapeutic, 53
Nursing homes, 25
Nyswander, M. E., 56

Occupational therapy, 22
Office of Child Development, 198
Office of Economic Opportunity, 194
Office of Education, 198
Old age

community mental health centers and,
98–100
deprivations in, 98
group psychotherapy in, 97
negative attitudes toward, 96–97
organic brain syndrome in, 97
positive approach to, 97–102
prospects in, 102–103
psychiatric needs of, 91–103
rehabilitation potential in, 96
service deficiency to, 98
society and, 102
see also Aged
Old-age assistance and insurance, 93
Operant conditioning, 21

Pacific Presbyterian Hospital, 34
Paraprofessionals
in children's mental health services, 106,
109, 114
in community mental health centers, 59,
201
education and, 114
Paris
district psychiatry in, 69–87
Institute of Psychoanalysis in, 72
Pasamanick, B., 4
Patients, "dumping" of, 37
Paumelle, Philippe, 69–87
Perceptual isolation, 5
Pettigrew, T. E., 214
Philadelphia, children's services in,
106–107
Phoenix House, drug abuse and, 139, 158
Piaget, J., 210
Powell v. Texas, 165
Preschool child preventive mental health,
112–113
developmental evaluation in, 113–114
President's Task Force on the Aging, 91,
94
President's Task Force on the Mentally
Handicapped, 94, 103
"Prevention syndrome," 187
Problem drinking, 167–168
see also Alocholism
Prochlorperazine (Compazine), alcoholism
and, 168

Prohibition era, 164
Project Re-Ed, 118
Psychiatric population explosion,
community center and, 46
Psychiatry
community, see Community psychiatry
old age and, 91–103
racism in, 222, 227
Psychoactive drugs, consciousness alteration
through, 129
Psychological cost-of-living index, 215
Psychopathology, age and, 92
Psychosis
community psychiatry and, 5–8
misconception of, 4
Psychotherapy
analytic-reconstructive, 20
behavior modification in, 21
deviant vs. adaptive behavior in, 21
milieu therapy and, 21
reeducative, 20
supportive, 20
Psychotic behavior
clinical description of, 19
integrative levels in, 19
Psychotic depression, chemotherapy in,
19–20
Psychotic patients, role of in community
mental health centers, 17
Psychotropic drugs, 5
Puget Sound Group Health Association,
195

Racism, in American psychiatry, 222, 227
Racism and Psychiatry (Thomas and
Sillen), 227
Recreation therapy, 22
Religion-oriented programs, drug abuse and,
'157–158
Revenue Sharing Act, 62
Riessman, F., 214
Robins, E., 175
Rogers, E. M., 214
Rousseau, Jean Jacques, 6

St. Elizabeths Hospital, 103
St. Mary's Hospital, 34
San Francisco, Westside Center in, 31–36

Saturday Review, 140

Scheid's cyanotic syndrome, 5

Schizophrenia
  in aged, 97
  deterioration in, 5
  as disuse atrophy in ego functions, 5

Schizophrenics
  day-hospital care for, 50–51
  effect of on community, 7
  family burden and, 6, 7 n.

Schizophrenic syndrome, iatrogenic features
    of, 5

Self-mutilation, 5

Senate Special Committee on Aging, 91
    103

Sheldon, E. B., 215

Sherif, M., 213

Singer Zone Center, 167

Skid row, 164

Skills, acquisitions of by children, 116–118

Sloate, Nathan, 91–103

Smith, R. L., 211

Social intervention, consequences of, 215

Sociotherapy, 21–22

Solomon, Harry C., 15

Somers, A. R., 202

Soundview-Throgs Neck Community
    Mental Health Center, 26–27

Soviet Union, community psychiatry in, 3

Staffing problems, community mental health
    centers, 57–58

Stinson, D., 174

Suicide Prevention, Inc., 32

Synanon, drug abuse and, 155

Teen Challenge, 157

Tertiary prevention, in drug abuse, 150–160

Therapeutic community, milieu therapy and,
    21

Therapeutic nursery school, 53

Thorazine, 168

Tranquilizers, alcoholism and, 176

Transcendental Meditation, 158

Trichotillomania, 5

Tuck, Jay Nelson, 178

Tuck, Lynne, 178

Uniform Alcoholism and Intoxication
    Treatment Act (1971), 165

Veterans Administration, 172

Warner, A., 56

Warren, Earl, 93

Watts (Los Angeles) Health Center,
    235–236

Welfare system, community mental health
    centers and, 191

Wellesley Human Relations Service, 234

Westchester Community Mental Health
    Board, 45, 61

Westchester County
    child-guidance clinic in, 43
    mental health services in, 62

West Philadelphia Mental Health
    Consortium, 186

Westside Community Mental Health
    Center, Inc. (San Francisco), 31–36,
    236–238
    computerized accountability system in, 35
    management information system in,
    35–36

White House Conference on the Aging, 91,
    103

Williamsbridge-Fordham mental health
    service, 28–29

Wolk, R. W., 97

Women alcoholics, 171

Woodlawn Organization, Chicago, 235

Work, in prevention of mental illness, 118

World Health Organization
    alcoholism and, 165
    drug use and, 131

World War II
    community mental health and, 69
    French poor and, 71

Zwerling, Israel, 15–29, 36–40